OXFORD MEDICAL PUBLICATIONS

# Pacemakers and ICDs

**Published and forthcoming Oxford Specialist Handbooks**

**General Oxford Specialist Handbooks**
A Resuscitation Room Guide (Banerjee and Hargreaves)

**Oxford Specialist Handbooks in End of Life Care**
Cardiology: From advanced disease to bereavement (Beattie, Connelly, and Watson eds.)
Nephrology: From advanced disease to bereavement (Brown, Chambers, and Eggeling)

**Oxford Specialist Handbooks in Anaesthesia**
Cardiac Anaesthesia (Barnard and Martin eds.)
Neuroanaesthesia (Nathanson and Moppett eds.)
Obstetric Anaesthesia (Clyburn, Collis, Harries, and Davies eds.)
Paediatric Anaesthesia (Doyle ed.)

**Oxford Specialist Handbooks in Cardiology**
Cardiac Catheterization and Coronary Angiography (Mitchell, Leeson, West, and Banning)
Pacemakers and ICDs (Timperley, Leeson, Mitchell, and Betts eds.)
Echocardiography (Leeson, Mitchell, and Becher eds.)
Heart Failure (Gardner, McDonagh and Walker)
Nuclear Cardiology (Sabharwal, Loong, and Kelion)

**Oxford Specialist Handbooks in Neurology**
Epilepsy (Alarcon, Nashef, Cross, and Nightingale)
Parkinson's Disease and Other Movement Disorders (Edwards, Bhatia, Quinn, and Swinn)

**Oxford Specialist Handbooks in Paediatrics**
Paediatric Gastroenterology, Hepatology, and Nutrition (Beattie, Dhawan, and Puntis eds.)
Paediatric Nephrology (Rees, Webb, and Brogan)
Paediatric Neurology (Forsyth and Newton eds.)
Paediatric Oncology and Haematology (Bailey and Skinner eds.)
Paediatric Radiology (Johnson, Williams, and Foster)

**Oxford Specialist Handbooks in Surgery**
Hand Surgery (Warwick)
Neurosurgery (Samandouras)
Otolaryngology and Head and Neck Surgery (Warner and Corbridge)
Plastic and Reconstructive Surgery (Giele and Cassell eds.)
Renal Transplantation (Talbot)
Urological Surgery (Reynard, Sullivan, Turner, Feneley, Armenakas, and Mark eds.)
Vascular Surgery (Hands, Murphy, Sharp, and Ray-Chaudhuri eds.)

# OXFORD

UNIVERSITY PRESS

Great Clarendon Street, Oxford OX2 6DP

Oxford University Press is a department of the University of Oxford.
It furthers the University's objective of excellence in research, scholarship,
and education by publishing worldwide in

Oxford New York

Auckland Cape Town Dar es Salaam Hong Kong Karachi
Kuala Lumpur Madrid Melbourne Mexico City Nairobi
New Delhi Shanghai Taipei Toronto

With offices in

Argentina Austria Brazil Chile Czech Republic France Greece
Guatemala Hungary Italy Japan Poland Portugal Singapore
South Korea Switzerland Thailand Turkey Ukraine Vietnam

Oxford is a registered trade mark of Oxford University Press
in the UK and in certain other countries

Published in the United States
by Oxford University Press Inc., New York

© Oxford University Press, 2008

The moral rights of the authors have been asserted
Database right Oxford University Press (maker)

First published 2008

British Library Cataloguing in Publication Data

Data available

Library of Congress Cataloging in Publication Data

Data available

Typeset by Newgen Imaging Systems (P) Ltd., Chennai, India
Printed in Italy
on acid-free paper by
LegoPrint S.p.A.

ISBN 978-0-19-857132-2 (flexicover: alk. paper)

10 9 8 7 6 5 4 3 2 1

Oxford University Press makes no representation, express or implied, that the drug
dosages in this book are correct. Readers must therefore always check the product
information and clinical procedures with the most up-to-date published product
information and data sheets provided by the manufacturers and the most recent
codes of conduct and safety regulations. The authors and the publishers do not
accept responsibility or legal liability for any errors in the text or for the misuse or
misapplication of material in this work. Except where otherwise stated, drug dosages
and recommendations are for the non-pregnant adult who is not breast-feeding.

# Oxford Specialist Handbooks in Cardiology

# Pacemakers and ICDs

Edited by

**Jonathan Timperley**
Specialist Registrar in Cardiology,
John Radcliffe Hospital,
Oxford, UK

**Paul Leeson**
Honorary Consultant Cardiologist,
John Radcliffe Hospital, Oxford, and
BHF Clinical Science Fellow,
University of Oxford, UK

**Andrew RJ Mitchell**
Consultant Cardiologist,
Jersey General Hospital, Jersey, Channel Islands and
Honorary Consultant Cardiologist,
John Radcliffe Hospital, Oxford, UK

and

**Timothy Betts**
Consultant Electrophysiologist
John Radcliffe Hospital,
Oxford, UK

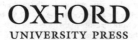

OXFORD
UNIVERSITY PRESS

# Foreword

This is a welcome addition to the Oxford Handbook Series. As usual in this series the advice is down to earth and very practical. The book is written by a team of contributors from the John Radcliffe Hospital in Oxford, although two are now consultant cardiologists in Southampton. In addition to the consultants the team includes specialist registrars and an ICD nurse specialist, some of whom have taken the lead on major sections of the book. One specialist registrars and three consultants have edited the book. This blend of talent and experience, which accurately reflects the range of work undertaken by an ICD/Pacing unit, is essential for such a practical and technical book which is intended to be read by a similarly wide range of professionals.

The illustrations are simple line drawings with a smattering of photographs and reproduced ECGs/electrograms. The timing cycles are consistently drawn and are an invaluable aid to the understanding of pacemaker function. There are good quality X-rays and fluoroscopy screen shots which are helpful to those who will use this book as a practical guide to providing a Pacing/ICD service. The subject of the book is largely technical and is not concerned with the evidence base from which stem the recommendations with regard to indications or pacing system choice, although a little history is given largely to add perspective rather than to inform a discussion on the merits of device selection for specific indications.

The content of this book concerns the whole range of rhythm management devices: pacemakers, implantable cardioverter defibrillators (ICDs), cardiac resynchronization therapy (CRT), usually with bi-ventricular (Bi-V) pacing), and combinations such as dual chamber or Bi-V ICDs (CRT-D). Implantable loop recorders (ILRs) are also covered in detail, which is relatively unusual but very welcome in a book of this sort.

There are many guidelines which have been published to assist the choice of device indication, selection of pacing mode, type of follow up, level of competence of staff, etc. Of these, the most comprehensive guidelines with the widest geographical authority are those that are constructed and published by the European Society of Cardiology, the American Heart Association, and the American College of Cardiology. Several agreed guidelines from all three of these professional societies are available in this area and it is these guidelines on which the authors most rely. This is fitting for a book which is designed to be valuable at an international level.

The utilization of implantable devices differs greatly from country to country and from district to district. Nothing could illustrate this better than the latest Eucomed figures for Europe (international comparisons) and the results of the *Pacemakers and Implantable Defibrillators: A Two Year National Survey for 2003 and 2004* carried out in the United Kingdom by the Network Devices Survey Group. The European data demonstrate that utilization of these implantable therapies is consistently far less than in the United States of America, and that there is very wide variation in the use of pacemakers, ICDs, and CRT devices which is not closely related to national wealth. The UK information, which is now being collected on a regular basis, shows that modest national implantation targets are not generally being met, and that there is enormous variability between device utilization across the country which probably reflects the concentration of trained electrophysiologists in the various health districts. The so-called 'postcode lottery' in this case is not directly related to finance but is probably due to a shortage of trained medical, nursing, and physiology staff. This book will provide the information base to assist the training of staff in these areas and as such it is most welcome.

This is a concise and helpful practical handbook for those charged with providing or contributing to a pacing, ICD, and ILR service. The origin of the book predominantly from a single centre and its reliance on accepted international guidelines give the book a consistent uniformity and an undisputed authority. The authors should be congratulated.

Professor John Camm
Professor of Clinical Cardiology
St. George's University of London
UK

# Preface

From the earliest days of pacemakers there has been a rapid advance in both the technology and ease of implantation of cardiac rhythm devices. Indications have expanded, implant numbers have soared, and device therapy now encompasses treatment of tachyarrhythmias with ICDs and heart failure with CRT. Device management is no longer the preserve of specialist tertiary centres.

This handbook is not designed to be a fully comprehensive manual of all current pacemakers and defibrillators; rather it is a practical book that explains concepts, principles, and a systematic approach to implantation, programming, and follow-up. It is as ideally suited to the cardiology trainee undergoing training on implantation as to the technician assisting at implantation and follow-up. It will also act as an easily accessible reference in times of need. Incorporating hints and tips from experts in the field, the familiar Oxford Handbook style, and clear diagrams and illustrations, we expect that this guide will become the standard for helping with implantation, follow-up, and troubleshooting for most implantable device procedures.

JT
PL
ARJM
TB
April 2007

# Acknowledgement

We would like to express our sincere thanks to the many individuals who read the text during its preparation and gave advice on its development.

# Contents

# Detailed contents

# Contributors

All chapters were edited by Jonathan Timperley, Paul Leeson, Andrew Mitchell, and Timothy Betts.

**Yaver Bashir**
Consultant Electrophysiologist,
John Radcliffe Hospital, Oxford
*Chapter 17: Perioperative
management of devices*

**Timothy Betts**
Consultant Electrophysiologist,
John Radcliffe Hospital, Oxford
*Chapter 5: Pacemaker programming
and device interrogation*
*Chapter 6: Troubleshooting
pacemakers*
*Chapter 12: Troubleshooting ICDs*

**Paul Leeson**
Specialist Registrar in Cardiology,
John Radcliffe Hospital, Oxford
*Chapter 1: Pacemaker principles*

**Nicola Meldrum**
ICD Nurse Specialist,
John Radcliffe Hospital, Oxford
*Chapter 15: Device clinic and
follow-up*

**Oliver Ormerod**
Consultant Cardiologist,
John Radcliffe Hospital, Oxford
*Chapter 2: Permanent pacemaker
implantation*

**Paul Roberts**
Consultant Electrophysiologist,
Southampton University Hospital
*Chapter 13: Cardiac
resynchronization therapy*

**Alisdair Ryding**
Specialist Registrar in Cardiology,
John Radcliffe Hospital, Oxford
*Chapter 8: Insertable loop
recorder*

**Jonathan Timperley**
Honorary Consultant Cardiologist,
John Radcliffe Hospital, Oxford
*Chapter 3: Pulse generator
replacement*
*Chapter 4: Pacemaker
complications*
*Chapter 7: Temporary cardiac
pacing*
*Chapter 9: ICD principles*
*Chapter 10: ICD implantation*
*Chapter 11: ICD programming*
*Chapter 16: Lifestyle issues,
patients' concerns, and devices*

**David Tomlinson**
Specialist Registrar in Cardiology,
John Radcliffe Hospital, Oxford
*Chapter 9: ICD principles*
*Chapter 10: ICD implantation*

**Arthur Yue**
Consultant Electrophysiologist,
Southampton University Hospital
*Chapter 14: System and lead
extractions*

# Useful websites

American Heart Association: *http://www.americanheart.org/*

American College of Cardiology: *http://www.acc.org/*

Arrhythmia Alliance: *http://www.arrhythmiaalliance.org.uk*

Biotronik: *http://www.biotronik.com*

British Cardiovascular Society: *http://www.bcs.com/*

British Heart Foundation: *http://www.bhf.org.uk/*

Driver and Vehicle Licensing Agency: *http://www.dvla.gov.uk/*

European Society of Cardiology *http://www.escardio.org/*

Guidant: *http://www.guidant.com*

Heart Rhythm Society: *http://www.hrsonline.org*

Heart Rhythm UK: *http://www.hruk.org.uk*

Medtronic: *http://www.medtronic.com*

National Institute for Clinical Excellence: *http://www.nice.org.uk*

Sorin Group: *http://www.elamedical.com*

St Jude Medical: *http://www.sjm.com*

# Symbols and abbreviations

| | |
|---|---|
| 📖 | cross-reference |
| 1° | primary |
| 2° | secondary |
| ABP | atrial blanking period |
| ACC | American College of Cardiology |
| AEI | atrial escape interval |
| AF | atrial fibrillation |
| AHA | American Heart Association |
| AMI | acute myocardial infarction |
| AP | anterior-posterior |
| ARP | atrial refractory period |
| ARVC | arrhythmogenic right ventricular cardiomyopathy |
| ASD | atrial septal defect |
| ATP | anti-tachycardia pacing |
| AV | atrioventricular |
| AVI | atrioventricular interval |
| AVN | atrioventricular node |
| BNP | brain natriuretic peptide |
| BOL | beginning of life |
| BiV | biventricular |
| CABG | coronary artery bypass grafting |
| CHF | congestive heart failure |
| CL | cycle length |
| CO | cardiac output |
| CPR | cardiopulmonary resuscitation |
| CRP | C-reactive protein |
| CRT | cardiac resynchronization therapy |
| CRT-D | cardiac resynchronization therapy defibrillator |
| CRT-P | cardiac resynchronization therapy pacemaker |
| CS | coronary sinus |
| CW | continuous wave (Doppler) |
| CXR | chest X-ray |
| DFT | defibrillation threshold |
| ECG | electrocardiogram |
| EF | ejection fraction |
| EGM | electrogram |

| | |
|---|---|
| EOL | end of life |
| EF | ejection fraction |
| EMI | electromagnetic interference |
| EPS | electrophysiological study |
| ERI | elective replacement indicator |
| ESC | European Society of Cardiology |
| ESR | erythrocyte sedimentation rate |
| FBC | full blood count |
| FVT | fast ventricular tachycardia |
| GA | general anaesthesia |
| HCM | hypertrophic cardiomyopathy |
| ICD | implantable cardioverter defibrillator |
| ILR | insertable loop recorder |
| INR | international normalized ratio |
| IV | intravenous |
| IVC | inferior vena cava |
| LA | left atrium |
| LAO | left anterior oblique |
| LAHB | left anterior hemiblock |
| LBBB | left bundle branch block |
| LPHB | left posterior hemiblock |
| LRI | lower rate interval |
| LRL | lower rate limit |
| LV | left ventricle |
| LVEDD | left ventricular end diastolic diameter |
| LVEF | left ventricular ejection fraction |
| LVESD | left ventricular end systolic diameter |
| LVOT | left ventricular outflow tract |
| MAP | mean arterial pressure |
| M, C, & S | microscopy, culture, and sensitivity |
| MD | morphology discriminator |
| MHRA | Medicines and Healthcare Products Regulatory Agency |
| MI | myocardial infarction |
| MR | mitral regurgitation |
| MRI | magnetic resonance imaging |
| MSDR | maximum sensor driven rate |
| MTR | maximum tracking rate |
| NASPE | North American Society for Pacing and Electrophysiology |
| NCAP | non-competitive atrial pacing |
| NCS | neurocardiogenic syncope |
| NICE | National Institution of Clinical Excellence |

| | |
|---|---|
| NID | number of intervals for detection |
| NSVT | non-sustained ventricular tachycardia |
| NYHA | New York Heart Association |
| PAC | premature atrial contraction |
| PAF | paroxysmal atrial fibrillation |
| pAVI | paced atrioventricular interval |
| PCI | percutaneous coronary intervention |
| PES | programmed electrical stimulation |
| PFO | patent foramen ovale |
| PAVB | post atrial ventricular blanking |
| PMT | pacemaker-mediated tachycardia |
| PSA | pacing system analyser |
| PVAB | post ventricular atrial blanking |
| PVARP | post-ventricular atrial refractory period |
| PVC | premature ventricular complex |
| PVS | programmed ventricular stimulation |
| PW | pulsed wave (Doppler) |
| QOL | quality of life |
| RA | right atrium |
| RAO | right anterior oblique |
| RDR | rate drop response |
| RBBB | right bundle branch block |
| RV | right ventricle |
| RVOT | right ventricular outflow tract |
| SAN | sinoatrial node |
| sAVI | sensed atrioventricular interval |
| SCD | sudden cardiac death |
| SDAEI | sensor driven atrial escape interval |
| SDI | sensor driven interval |
| SRD | sustained rate duration |
| SVC | superior vena cava |
| SVT | supraventricular tachycardia |
| TARP | total atrial refractory period |
| TB | tuberculosis |
| TDI | tissue Doppler imaging |
| TOE | transoesophageal echocardiography |
| U & E | urea and electrolytes |
| URI | upper rate interval |
| URL | upper rate limit |
| VBP | ventricular blanking period |
| VF | ventricular fibrillation |

| VO$_2$ | oxygen consumption |
|---|---|
| VRP | ventricular refractory period |
| VSD | ventricular septal defect |
| VSP | ventricular safety pacing |
| VT | ventricular tachycardia |
| VTC | vector timing and correlation |
| WPW | Wolff–Parkinson–White (syndrome) |

# Pacemaker principles

# History of devices

## Pacemakers

Since their first use, well over 2 million pacemakers have been implanted worldwide. The first artificial pacemaker was an external device designed and built in 1950 by John Hopps. The first totally internal device was implanted into a patient in 1958 by Elmqvist and Senning from Sweden. The patient, Arne Larson, suffered with Stokes–Adams attacks following a viral myocarditis leading to complete heart block. His first device lasted only a few hours before the battery leaked acid into the epoxy casing. The second device lasted for 6 weeks. Mr. Larson eventually died at the age of 86 having received a total of 23 device implants.

Initial internal devices used zinc–mercury batteries, which were prone to leaking. They soon improved with changes to the original design including welded connections between the inner and outer cans and improved double wrap separators. In the late 1970s lithium batteries became standard and resulted in greatly extended battery life.

The first systems relied on surgically placed epicardial leads. The first endocardial systems were implanted in the 1960s. Initial devices were 'fixed rate'. 'Demand' pacemakers were also introduced in the mid-1960s. During subsequent years there were advances in lead and device design, leading to smaller pacemakers with longer battery life and with more advanced diagnostic features.

## Implantable defibrillators

Despite a large amount of scepticism (even from within the cardiology community), the first implantable cardioverter defibrillator (ICD) was developed by Michel Mirowski's team and implanted in 1980. There have now been over 65,000 patients treated with this form of therapy. Initial systems were large and required a thoracotomy with epicardial electrode positioning. The device was implanted in the abdominal wall. Mirroring the advances in pacemakers, advances in electronics, battery and lead technology resulted in the first transvenous system implanted prepectorally in 1995.

## Cardiac resynchronization therapy

The interest in pacing the left ventricle for haemodynamic reasons began in the early 1990s. Following on from initial systems using epicardial electrodes implanted surgically, transvenous systems pacing the left ventricle via the coronary sinus transformed this type of therapy. Initially a Y-connector to the right ventricle (RV) port of a standard dual chamber pacemaker was used. This approach was followed by devices with a dedicated left ventricle (LV) port allowing for separate timings and outputs to the RV and LV channels.

## Timeline of devices

| 1957 | First transistorized, battery-powered wearable pacemaker |
| 1960 | First totally implanted system |
| 1962 | First endocardial pacing lead |
| 1969 | First 'demand' pacemaker |
| 1975 | Introduction of the lithium iodine battery |
| 1980 | First ICD inserted |
| 1988 | First rate-responsive pacemaker |
| 1994 | First demonstration of potential benefits of multisite pacing |
| 1995 | First prepectoral ICD |
| 2001 | First combined CRT and ICD device (CRT-D) |

# Anatomy of the conducting system

The conduction system of the heart (Fig. 1.1) generates coordinated waves of electrical activity that pass sequentially through the atria and ventricles. The system is required to have an intrinsic ability to generate impulses and direct them through the myocardium. Impulses are generated in the sinoatrial node (SAN), travel in the longitudinal direction of atrial muscle fibres and then converge on the atrioventricular (AV) node. From the AV node they are funnelled through the His bundle and spread out through the ventricles via the branch bundles. They are delivered to the myocardium by the Purkinje fibres.

**Sinoatrial node** The SAN is a distinct structure lying within the epicardium at the junction of the superior vena cava and right atrium. It is composed of P cells (which have an intrinsic ability to initiate impulses) and transitional cells (which morphologically lie between P cells and atrial myocardium) held within a collagen framework. Conduction fibres extend through the node into the atrium. The node has an autonomic nervous supply and its own arterial branch (the sinoatrial nodal artery) that arises from the right coronary artery in around 55% of people and the left circumflex in 45%.

**Atrioventricular node** The AV node is a less clearly defined subendocardial structure lying within the atrial septum. Anatomically it is located at the apex of *Koch*, the borders of which are the coronary sinus os, the tendon of *Todaro* and the septal leaflet of the tricuspid valve. It is more loosely composed than the sinus node and contains a variety of atrial, transitional, P, and conduction cells within a collagen network. It has an autonomic nervous supply and its own arterial branch (the AV nodal artery) that arises from the right coronary artery in around 90% of people (left circumflex in the remainder).

**His bundle** The His bundle joins the AV node to the bundle branches and lies within the membranous septum. It is a tubular bundle of parallel conduction fibres within a collagenous framework. It has minimal nervous supply but arterial supply from the AV nodal artery and septal branches of the left anterior descending artery.

**Bundle branches** The bundle branches extend from the His bundle through the ventricles. There is significant interindividual variation in the arrangement of these ventricular conduction fibres. However, there is classically a right bundle that extends down the right side of the interventricular septum and a large left bundle that spreads through the left ventricle as two or three distinct tracts. The bundle branches end in the Purkinje network that delivers the electrical impulses to the myocardium. There is minimal autonomic supply but extensive blood supply from all coronary arteries.

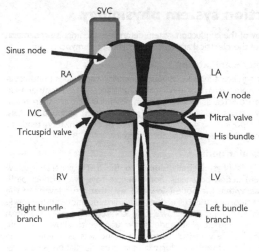

**Fig. 1.1** Anatomy of conducting system.

# Conduction system physiology

The physiology of the conduction system determines the impulse generation and transfer of the electrical activation throughout the myocardium.

## Sinoatrial node and atrium

The SAN has significant intrinsic impulse generation capabilities (automaticity) and is the main pacemaker in normal circumstances. The sinoatrial node cells generate slow (calcium-driven) action potentials that are then transferred rapidly across the atria via fast (sodium-driven) action potentials. Because of the position of the node the wave of depolarization tends to travel through both atria from superior to inferior.

## Atrioventricular node

The AV node is physiologically similar to the SAN, generating slow (calcium-driven) action potentials. Some people have two distinct pathways, or areas, within the node (slow and fast) that are relevant to the generation of supraventricular arrhythmias. The position of the node between atria and ventricles allows it to control passage of electrical impulses to the ventricle. The node delays transfer to allow complete atrial emptying before ventricular contraction and acts as a limit on the rate of ventricular activation in, for example, atrial fibrillation. The node also has some intrinsic automaticity that allows impulse generation.

## His bundle and bundle branches

The His bundle has distinct longitudinal fibres that direct electrical impulses to the ventricles. The bundle branches are direct continuations of these fibres. The *His-Purkinje* system facilitates rapid global depolarization through the ventricles, typically producing a narrow QRS complex on the surface ECG.

## Anatomy of the venous system

# Anatomy of the venous system

Venous access for permanent pacing is usually via the subclavian, cephalic, or axillary veins and for temporary pacing via the subclavian, internal jugular, or femoral veins. See Fig. 1.2.

**Cephalic vein** This is a superficial vein starting from the dorsal venous network of the hand that winds up the radial side of the forearm, over the elbow to the lateral border of biceps. It then passes between the pectoralis major and deltoid muscles in the *delto-pectoral groove* (the access site for pacing). The cephalic vein then joins the axillary vein just below the clavicle.

**Axillary vein** This is an upper limb deep vein starting as a continuation of the basilic vein at the lower border of teres major. It joins the cephalic vein to form the subclavian vein at the lateral border of the first rib after the cephalic vein.

**Subclavian vein** This extends to the sternal end of the clavicle where it joins the internal jugular to form the innominate vein. It lies in a groove on the surface of the first rib and pleura where it is accessed for pacing. It has valves around 2cm from its end.

**Internal jugular vein** This originates at the base of the skull and drains vertically, lateral to the internal carotid artery and common carotid artery, before joining the subclavian veins to form the innominate veins. Access is usually in the triangle formed by sternal and clavicular heads of sternocleidomastoid.

**Innominate vein** The right vein is short and passes directly downwards to join the left innominate (a longer vessel passing obliquely across the chest) below the first rib by the right side of the sternum. They join to form the superior vena cava.

**Superior vena cava** This empties into the right atrium. A *persistent left superior vena cava* is sometimes found. In this situation the venous drainage on the right is normal via a superior vena cava-like structure to the right atrium but there is a separate left-sided drainage, usually to the coronary sinus.

**Femoral vein** The femoral vein accompanies the femoral artery through the upper two-thirds of the thigh. By the inguinal ligament it lies medial to the artery. The vein continues as the external iliac at the inguinal ligament and joins the hypogastric vein to form the common iliac vein.

**Inferior vena cava** The inferior vena cava is formed by the union of the left and right common iliac veins usually around the level of the fifth lumbar vertebra. It travels upwards and enters the inferior aspect of the right atrium.

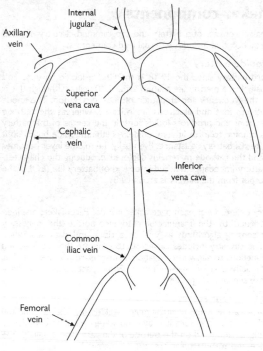

**Fig. 1.2** Anatomy of the venous system.

# Pacemaker components

The pacemaker consists of a battery and programmed circuitry encased within a metal box that includes external lead connectors.

## Lithium iodide battery

The standard battery since the 1970s is the lithium iodide battery. This battery usually has a median life span of around 10 years, although this is affected by the frequency and amplitude of pulse generation. The anode produces lithium ions and electrons are released, whereas the cathode collects electrons and produces iodide ions. In the centre of the battery these ions combine to form lithium iodide. As lithium iodide builds up it increases internal battery resistance. Eventually the middle layer becomes very thick and the cathode material is depleted, producing the characteristic high battery impedance that indicates end of battery life (EOL). The standard output from the battery is around 2.8V.

## Circuitry

The circuitry defines what each pacemaker can do. Pacemakers are individually designed by the manufacturer to incorporate the necessary pacing and sensing algorithms as well as a clock and data acquisition functions. The circuitry includes capacitors to generate the impulses and telemetry functions to allow interrogation. A magnet-responsive switch is included for activation of 'magnet mode'. Some pacemakers also have rate response sensors (□ p. 108).

## Case and lead connectors

The generator case is made of titanium and welded together around the battery and circuitry to ensure it is air- and watertight. The connectors are epoxy plastic and fixed on the outside of the case. The details of the pacing device and manufacturer are usually engraved on the outside of the case. The lead connectors are also usually labelled to ensure they are connected correctly.

## Battery indicators
- EOL: end of life (basic pacemaker functions no longer work).
- ERI: elective replacement indicator (the battery voltage is depleted and close to EOL. Generator replacement should be performed within 2–3 months).

Pacemakers may exhibit diagnostic ERI characteristics when the battery is nearly depleted. These include:
- a fixed decrease in the magnet rate (the rate the pacemaker switches to when a magnet is held over it);
- an increase in the pulse width to compensate for the lower voltage output;
- change to a simpler pacing mode, e.g. DDDR to VVI or VOO to reduce battery current drain.

## How to increase battery life
- Minimize the amount of pacing required
- Use pulses with a smaller voltage amplitude.
- Use pulses with a shorter duration.
- Use automated capture function (□ p. 122).

# Pacing leads

Pacing leads are flexible insulated wires. They have two ends (the *electrode tip* and *connector pin*) joined by the *conductor*, which is surrounded by *insulation*. They also have some form of *fixation* mechanism at the tip.

## Electrode

The electrode tip usually has an irregular surface to maximize surface area (and optimize polarization for pacing) while maintaining a small radius (to increase current density for pacing). The tips also need to be biologically inert and not degrade. They may be coated with microspheres or metallic meshes to create these characteristics. A common structure is to have a combination of titanium and platinum. Carbon elements can also be used. *Steroid eluting tips* incorporate a steroid, often impregnated in a silicone core. The steroid elutes from the tip and reduces inflammation, stabilizing and improving pacing thresholds over time. Single-pass VDD (📖 p. 24) leads, which are standard ventricular leads with two additional ring electrodes more proximally on the lead in the right atrium allowing for atrial sensing (but not pacing), are available.

## Fixation

There are two types of fixation—active and passive. Passive leads usually have small *tines* at the end (similar to soft 'fish hooks') that hold in the myocardial trabeculae. Active fixation leads have a screw mechanism in the end. These may be a fixed screw that requires the whole lead to be screwed in, but more commonly the screw is advanced from the tip by twisting of a central wire. This also simplifies screw retraction if a lead explant is required.

## Conductor and insulation

The conductor needs to be flexible, strong, and to have minimal current loss along its length. Conductors usually consist of multiple nickel-alloy wires, wound together. Unipolar wires have a single conductor and bipolar leads have a coaxial (with the distal electrode in the centre and the more proximal electrode wrapped around the outside) or a side-by-side design. The insulation is usually silicone rubber or a type of polyurethane.

## Connectors

The connector is a metallic pin with one or two separate junctions depending on whether the lead is uni- or bipolar. Around the connector there are sealing rings to ensure it fits snugly into the generator head. There is now an internationally agreed connector design to allow leads from one manufacturer to be fitted to a generator from another. This is known as IS-1. Originally, however, there was significant variation in design between manufacturers. Problems can still occasionally occur during generator replacement of older systems. Prior knowledge of the implanted leads is required to ensure the correct adaptor is available.

## Types of leads

### Unipolar pacing leads

*Unipolar pacing leads* have a single wire core and electrode tip. The pacemaker generator (the 'can') acts as the other electrode. The pacing and sensing circuit therefore travels through the body from the can to the tip of the pacing lead and then back to the pacemaker can through the lead (or the other way around, depending upon the programmed polarities of the electrode and can). As the current travels through the body, the surface ECG records a large pacing spike.

### Bipolar pacing leads (Fig. 1.3)

In a *bipolar pacing lead* there are two inner wire cores, separated by insulation, with two separate electrodes—one at the tip of the lead (tip electrode) and the other usually a few mm behind it (ring electrode). The pacing and sensing circuit travels down one inner wire from the can to the tip, crosses a few mm of myocardium to the ring electrode, and travels back to the can via the other inner wire. The surface ECG registers a much smaller pacing spike.

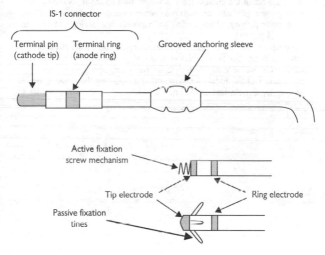

**Fig. 1.3** Pacing lead components of bipolar leads.

# Sensing

A pacemaker does not sense the surface ECG. It senses the potential difference between two electrodes: usually the *distal tip* and the *proximal ring electrode* in a bipolar lead or the *distal tip* and *pacemaker can* in a unipolar lead. The voltage difference produces an *intracardiac electrogram*.

The timing of the electrogram (EGM) represents local depolarization at the tip of the pacing electrode. Typically, the right ventricular lead tip is positioned at the apex of the right ventricle, which may be some distance from the area of earliest ventricular depolarization (distal right bundle branch). Therefore the EGM occurs a short time after the onset of the QRS complex on the surface ECG.

## Pacing sensitivity

Sensitivity can be programmed. The value represents the minimum local EGM amplitude that is registered as a sensed event. Any EGM component smaller than the programmed sensitivity is ignored.

- The ideal sensitivity will result in appropriate detection of intrinsic events (atrial or ventricular depolarization) with a large safety margin in case the amplitude of the local EGM decreases, e.g. ectopic beats, or, in the atrium, a change from sinus rhythm to atrial fibrillation.
- Setting the sensitivity too high may result in *undersensing* of atrial or ventricular activity, often leading to inappropriate pacing or failure to track (📖 p. 144).
- If the pacemaker is *oversensitive* then spurious electrical activation may result in inappropriate inhibition or tracking. The most common scenario is oversensing of ventricular repolarization (the T-wave component of the local electrogram) and counting this as another ventricular depolarization (📖 p. 138).

## Confusion over sensitivity (Fig. 1.4)

People easily become confused over what it means to *increase* or *decrease* sensitivity. Even if the operator understands, an instruction to an assistant to 'increase sensitivity' can lead to mistakes. This is because an *increase* in the 'value on the dial' of the pacemaker leads to a *decrease* in the number of events being sensed. If you want to make a pacemaker *less sensitive* the implication is that you want it to sense fewer events. However, this is achieved by an *increase* in the *sensitivity* (the 'value on the pacemaker dial') as this *increases* the minimum voltage level required for an event to be a sensed. *Sensitivity* is quantitative and defines the voltage level at which events start to be sensed. How *sensitive* a pacemaker is is qualitative and to make it less sensitive you increase the sensitivity.

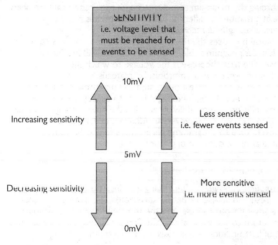

**Fig. 1.4** Sensitivity.

# Pacing

The pacemaker generates a pulse at a specific voltage for a defined period of time (pulse duration) by a capacitor discharge. The capacitor is charged from the battery and, as battery output is around 2.8V, higher pacing stimuli require simultaneous charging and discharge of two or three parallel capacitors (thereby shortening battery life).

## Threshold

- The *pacing threshold* (Fig. 1.5) is expressed in terms of the voltage and pulse duration and represents the smallest output voltage or shortest pulse duration required to initiate a depolarization wavefront. Either the pulse duration is fixed (e.g. at 0.5ms) and the voltage reduced stepwise to determine the minimum voltage required for capture or the voltage may be kept constant (e.g. 1mV) and the shortest pulse duration required for capture is then determined.
- By recording the minimum stimulus strength required to capture heart muscle at a number of different pulse durations, it is possible to construct a *strength–duration curve*. (Fig. 1.6.)
- For practical purposes the *rheobase* is the minimum stimulus strength at the longest programmable pulse duration that will produce a response. The true rheobase is the voltage to which the strength–duration curve asymptotes, i.e. plateaus.
- The *chronaxie* is the shortest pulse duration that produces a response when the stimulus strength (voltage) is set to exactly 2 × the *rheobase*.
- The most efficient energy delivery is when the pulse duration is equal to the *chronaxie* value. However, an adequate safety margin is required. It is conventional to programme pacemakers to 2 × the voltage threshold at pulse duration of 0.4 or 0.5ms.

## Pacing threshold evolution

During the first 2–4 weeks after pacing lead insertion, inflammation and oedema result in a rise in pacing threshold. This gradually resolves, leaving a small fibrous capsule, and the threshold decreases, although it may not return to the value at implant. Steroid eluting leads reduce the amount of inflammation and fibrosis and minimize these changes.

## High impedance leads

High impedance leads have a small electrode surface area in contact with the myocardium and a greater current density, resulting in more favourable thresholds. Higher impedances also result in decreased current drain and longer battery life.

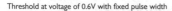

Threshold at voltage of 0.6V with fixed pulse width

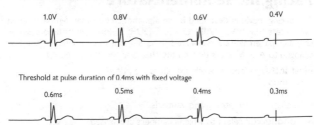

1.0V    0.8V    0.6V    0.4V

Threshold at pulse duration of 0.4ms with fixed voltage

0.6ms    0.5ms    0.4ms    0.3ms

**Fig. 1.5** Ventricular pacing threshold. Note capture of ventricle is lost as the voltage (or pulse duration) is reduced.

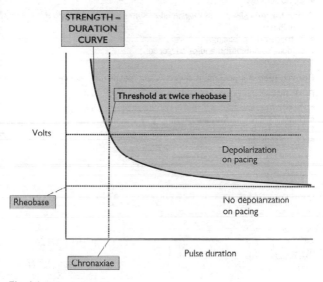

STRENGTH –
DURATION
CURVE

Threshold at twice rheobase

Volts

Depolarization
on pacing

Rheobase

No depolarization
on pacing

Pulse duration

Chronaxiae

**Fig. 1.6** Strength–duration curve.

# Pacing mode nomenclature

The pacing mode is described by an alphabetic code that can have up to five letters, e.g. VVI, AAIR, DDO, DDDR. Before implantation, single chamber pacemakers are referred to as SSI, but once implanted the S is changed to A or V depending on the chamber paced and sensed.

**First letter** refers to which chambers are *paced*.
- A, atrium.
- V, ventricle.
- D, dual, i.e. both atrium and ventricle.

**Second letter** refers to which chambers are *sensed*.
- A, atrium.
- V, ventricle.
- D, dual, i.e. both atrium and ventricle.
- O, no sensing.

**Third letter** refers to the *action* taken when an event is *sensed*.
- I, inhibition.
- T, triggered, i.e. pacing.
- D, dual, i.e. inhibition and/or triggered.
- O, no action.

**Fourth letter** if present, is always R and means *rate response*.

**Fifth letter** if present, indicates *multisite pacing*.
- A, atrium.
- V, ventricle.
- D, dual, i.e. both atrium and ventricle.
- O, no sensing.

# Pacemaker modes

### VOO (Fig. 1.7)

- Ventricular pacing.
- No sensing.
- No response to sensed events.

*Asynchronous, competitive pacing, 'magnet mode'*

The pacemaker paces the ventricle with a fixed, pre-programmed lower rate interval (LRI) (📖 p. 96) ignoring any underlying intrinsic rhythm. Pacing spikes will occur at regular fixed intervals, regardless of whether there is a QRS complex before, during, or after the pacing spike.

If there is no underlying rhythm, each pacing spike is followed by a QRS complex. If there is a competing underlying rhythm and the pacing spike falls in the ventricular myocardium refractory period following an intrinsic beat, it will not capture and there will be no QRS complex following it. Should a pacing spike land on the T wave of an intrinsic beat there is a small possibility of ventricular pro-arrhythmia. This risk is more likely in the setting of severe electrolyte imbalance or myocardial ischaemia.

VOO mode is the default mode that occurs when a pacemaker magnet is positioned over the pulse generator (📖 p. 354).

### AOO (Fig. 1.8)

- Atrial pacing.
- No sensing.
- No response to sensed events.

*Atrial asynchronous pacing*

Similar to VOO mode but pacing only occurs in the atrial chamber. There is no sensing and no response to intrinsic events.

### DOO (Fig. 1.9)

- Dual chamber pacing.
- No sensing.
- No response to sensed events.

*Dual chamber or AV sequential asynchronous pacing*

Again, no sensing, but constant pacing stimuli delivered first to the atrium and then, after a fixed AV delay, to the ventricle. The intervals never change.

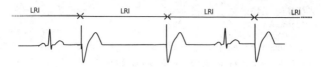

**Fig. 1.7** VOO pacing. Fixed rate ventricular pacing at lower rate interval (LRI) irrespective of underlying atrial or ventricular activity.

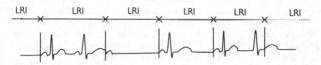

**Fig. 1.8** AOO pacing. Fixed rate atrial pacing at LRI irrespective of underlying atrial or ventricular activity.

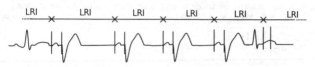

**Fig. 1.9** DOO pacing. Fixed rate atrial and ventricular pacing at LRI irrespective of underlying atrial or ventricular activity.

### VVI (Fig. 1.10)
- Ventricular pacing.
- Ventricular sensing.
- Inhibited ventricular pacing if ventricular impulse sensed.

#### Ventricular demand pacing, ventricular inhibited pacing
A minimum ventricular rate is programmed that determines the maximum interval allowed between consecutive ventricular beats, either intrinsic or paced (e.g. 60bpm or 1000ms intervals) and determines the lower rate limit (LRL) (📖 p. 96).

With a LRL of 60bpm, following a sensed or paced ventricular beat, the pacemaker clock starts counting up to 1000ms. If there is no sensed event by the time it reaches 1000ms a pacing impulse is delivered. If an intrinsic impulse is sensed before the pacemaker clock reaches 1000ms, any pacing is inhibited and the internal pacemaker clock is reset back to zero and starts counting up to 1000ms from the beginning.

There will be a programmable ventricular refractory period (VRP) (📖 p. 104) that follows a sensed or paced ventricular beat. During the VRP, sensed ventricular events are ignored and do not affect the timing cycles.

The ventricular rate should be no slower than the programmed bradycardia rate but may be faster if there is an intrinsic rhythm that is greater than the pacemaker bradycardia rate.

### AAI (Fig. 1.11)
- Atrial pacing.
- Atrial sensing.
- Inhibited atrial pacing if atrial impulse sensed.

#### Atrial demand pacing, atrial inhibited pacing
This is similar to VVI pacing but there is only pacing and sensing in the atrium. A sensed or paced atrial event initiates a refractory period during which any further sensed atrial events are ignored. As with VVI pacing, there is a LRI, which is the maximum time allowed between successive atrial events. If there are no sensed events during the LRI an atrial paced complex will occur at the end of the LRI.

### DVI (Fig. 1.12)
- Dual chamber pacing.
- Ventricular sensing.
- Inhibition of ventricular pacing if there is a sensed ventricular event.

#### AV sequential, ventricular inhibited pacing
This is rarely used. Although the pacemaker may be inhibited and reset by ventricular events, all intrinsic atrial events are ignored and there is constant atrial pacing. Programmable parameters include an LRI, an atrioventricular interval (AVI, 📖 p. 100), and a VRP (📖 p. 104).

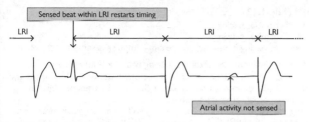

**Fig. 1.10** VVI pacing. Ventricular pacing and sensing.

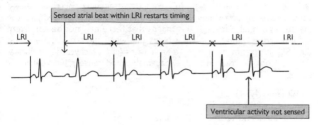

**Fig. 1.11** AAI pacing. Atrial pacing and sensing.

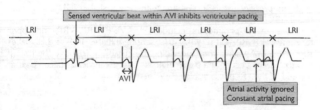

**Fig. 1.12** DVI pacing. Constant atrial pacing with ventricular pacing and inhibition.

### DDI (Fig. 1.13)
- Dual chamber pacing.
- Dual chamber sensing.
- Inhibited pacing in ventricle or atrium if impulse is sensed in chamber.

#### AV sequential, non-P synchronous pacing with dual-chamber sensing
This is essentially DDD pacing without atrial tracking. This means the paced ventricular rate cannot be faster than the programmed LRL, even if the sensed atrial rate exceeds this.

Programmable parameters include LRI, AVI, post-ventricular atrial refractory period (PVARP) (📖 p. 104), and VRP. If a P wave occurs after the PVARP and is sensed there is no atrial pacing (i.e. inhibition). The subsequent ventricular pacing spike cannot be delivered until the end of the VV interval, defined by the LRI. Atrial pacing occurs at the end of the atrial escape interval (📖 p. 96) from the preceding paced or sensed ventricular event, providing there is no inhibition from a sensed event in the atrial channel. Although this means that there may not be consistent AV synchrony when there is AV block (i.e. when the atrial rate exceeds the LRL), it does mean that rapid atrial rates (atrial tachycardia or fibrillation) will not be tracked by the pacemaker and cause rapid ventricular pacing.

### VDD (Fig. 1.14)
- Ventricular pacing.
- Dual (atrial and ventricular) sensing.
- Dual response (inhibition or triggering).

#### Atrial synchronous, P-tracking
Although this mode is an option in pacemakers with atrial and ventricular leads, its primary use is in systems with only a single VDD pacing lead (📖 p. 12).

Programmable parameters include LRI, AVI, PVARP, VRP, and upper rate interval (URI) (📖 p. 98). Atrial sensing initiates an AVI that makes sure there is AV synchrony, providing the atrial rate is above the LRL. If no atrial event occurs, the pacemaker initiates a ventricular paced beat at the end of the LRI (i.e. it displays 'VVI' activity.)

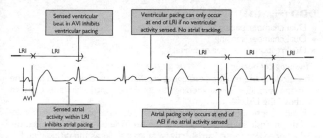

**Fig. 1.13** DDI pacing. Dual chamber pacing and sensing but no triggering of ventricular pacing in response to intrinsic atrial activity.

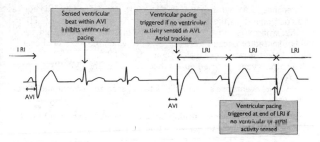

**Fig. 1.14** VDD pacing. Ventricular pacing with dual chamber sensing.

**DDD (Fig. 1.15)**
- Dual chamber pacing.
- Dual chamber sensing.
- Dual response (trigger or inhibit).

*'Physiological pacing'*

This mode is the most physiological, maintaining synchrony between the atria and ventricles whilst keeping the atrial and ventricular rates equal to or above the LRL.
- If the intrinsic sinus rate is less than the LRL, atrial pacing occurs.
- If the intrinsic sinus rate increases, the ventricle can track the speed of the underlying sensed atrial activity, at least as far as the rate defined by the programmed URI.
- Following atrial sensing or pacing, if ventricular activation does not occur by the end of the programmed AVI, there is ventricular pacing.

Maintenance of AV synchrony at or above the rate defined by LRI requires two components to the timing cycle, the atrial escape interval (AEI) and the AVI where the LRI = AEI + AVI. The AEI is the maximum time from the last sensed or paced ventricular event to when the next atrial event is due to keep the rate more than or equal to the LRL.
- If an atrial event is sensed during that time (after the PVARP) it initiates an AVI.
- If no atrial events are sensed, it initiates a paced atrial event and starts the AVI.

Programmable parameters include LRI, AVI, PVARP, VRP, and URI. The LRL can be either atrial or ventricular based (📖 p. 96).

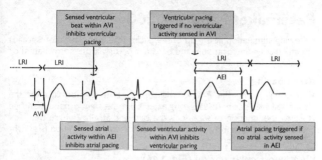

**Fig. 1.15** DDD pacing. Physiological pacing with ventricular pacing and inhibition.

# Pacemakers and the ECG

Following stimulation at the tip of the pacing lead, depolarization spreads directly through myocardium and does not occur via the normal atrial or specialized His–Purkinje conduction system.

## Atrial pacing

With atrial pacing the P-wave will appear relatively normal after the pacing spike as pacing usually originates from the right atrial appendage close to the junction of superior vena cava and atrium (where the SAN lies) and passes inferiorly. If the lead is in an alternative position (e.g. right atrial free wall) it may appear different.

## Right ventricular pacing (Fig. 1.16)

With a standard right ventricular pacing lead, ventricular depolarization starts in the right ventricle, spreads across the interventricular septum, and then spreads through the left ventricle. The paced QRS complex therefore usually resembles LBBB morphology (negative polarity in V1, positive polarity in V6).

## Left ventricular pacing (Fig. 1.16)

Pacing the left ventricle first means the left ventricle depolarizes before the right ventricle and the QRS complex therefore resembles RBBB morphology (positive polarity in V1, negative polarity in V6). Left ventricular pacing can be purposeful, i.e. deliberate left ventricular pacing with a left ventricular lead via the coronary sinus, or inadvertent due to a misplaced right ventricular pacing wire stimulating the left ventricle. This can occur if the lead passes through a patent foramen ovale, atrial septal defect, or ventricular septal defect or is placed in a coronary vein.

## Paced fusion and pseudofusion beats (Fig. 1.17)

With intrinsic conduction through the AV node, if the programmed AVI is longer than the intrinsic PR interval but shorter than the time taken for depolarization to reach the lead tip and be sensed, ventricular pacing will not be inhibited. A ventricular pacing spike is delivered from the right ventricular apex and fuses with the intrinsic QRS complex a *paced* fusion beat. The first part of the QRS complex resembles the underlying intrinsic QRS morphology, a pacing spike appears just after the onset of the QRS, and the remainder of the QRS is more broad and slurred. The overall QRS duration is between that of the intrinsic and fully paced QRS durations.

With *pseudofusion* the QRS is a native QRS with the addition of a pacing spike that, because of its timing, causes no depolarization.

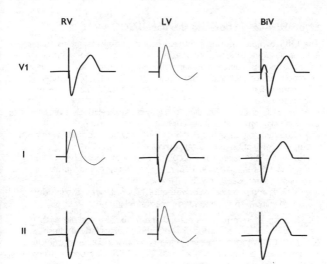

**Fig. 1.16** Right ventricular, left ventricular, and biventricular pacing.

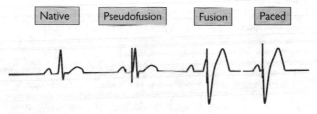

**Fig. 1.17** Native, pseudofusion, fusion, and paced beats.

## Myocardial infarction and the paced ECG

The QRS complex during right ventricular pacing resembles that of left bundle branch block. This means that the conventional criteria of ST elevation, ST depression, and T-wave inversion for myocardial infarction or ischaemia are not applicable. Likewise, the established ECG criteria for old myocardial infarction, such as Q waves, lose their diagnostic value.

A few ECG criteria, although not sensitive, are relatively specific for the diagnosis of myocardial infarction.

- A qR complex in leads I, aVL, V5, and V6 may be associated with an old, extensive anteroseptal myocardial infarction.
- Notching of the ascending limb of the S wave in at least two of V3 to V5 (Cabrera's sign; see Fig. 1.18) may also be associated with an old, extensive anteroseptal myocardial infarction.
- qR or QR complexes with or without Carbera's sign in the inferior leads may indicate old inferior myocardial infarction.

ST elevation > 5mm in predominantly negative QRS complexes is the best marker of acute myocardial infarction, particularly if there is a previous ECG without ST elevation for comparison. Other signs include ST depression ≥ 1mm in V1, V2, and V3 and ST elevation > 1mm in leads with a concordant QRS polarity.

## T-wave memory

Continuous ventricular pacing can result in the phenomenon of T-wave memory in which subsequent, intrinsically conducted native QRS complexes are followed by inverted T waves or, less commonly, ST segment abnormalities. These are a consequence of right ventricular pacing rather than ischaemia or infarction. The abnormal depolarization following right ventricular pacing results in persistent abnormal repolarization even during subsequent intrinsic beats. This is most commonly seen in the precordial and inferior leads. The T-wave polarity is in the same direction as the QRS polarity. Thus, inhibition of a pacemaker may allow accurate identification of pathological Q waves in underlying narrow complex beats, but ST-segment and T-wave changes cannot be interpreted reliably.

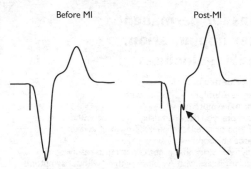

Before MI                    Post-MI

**Fig. 1.18** Cabrera's sign. During MI there may be subtle ECG changes, most easily recognized by comparing to a pre-MI ECG (left). Cabrera's sign (arrow) is a notched appearance on the ascending limb of the QRS seen in the precordial chest leads.

# Indications for permanent pacemaker implantation: AHA/ACC/ESC guidelines[1]

## Class I (good evidence)

- 2nd or 3rd degree AV block (📖 p. 38) with:
  - bradycardia and symptoms;
  - drug-induced bradycardia when drug cannot be withdrawn;
  - asystole of > 3s or rate less than 40bpm whilst awake;
  - after AV node ablation;
  - postoperative AV block that is not expected to resolve;
  - neuromuscular disease with AV block with or without symptoms.
- Patients with bifascicular or trifascicular block and:
  - intermittent 3rd degree AV block;
  - type II 2nd degree AV block;
  - alternating bundle branch block (📖 p. 38).
- Sinus node dysfunction (📖 p. 34) with symptomatic pauses.
- Symptomatic chronotropic incompetence (📖 p. 34).
- Pause-dependent ventricular tachycardia (VT) with or without prolonged QT (📖 p. 44).
- Recurrent syncope caused by carotid sinus hypersensitivity and a ventricular pause of > 3s (📖 p. 40).

## Class IIa/IIb (some evidence in favour)

- Asymptomatic 3rd degree AV block with escape rate > 40bpm.
- Asymptomatic type II 2nd degree AV block with a narrow complex QRS.
- 1st or 2nd degree AV block with symptoms similar to those of pacemaker syndrome.
- Asymptomatic sinus bradycardia < 40bpm.
- High risk patients with congenital long QT syndrome (📖 p. 44).
- Recurrent unprovoked syncope in patients with a hypersensitive cardioinhibitory response (📖 p. 40).
- Recurrent symptomatic neurocardiogenic syncope with bradycardia (📖 p. 40).

## Reference

1 ACC/AHA/NASPE (2002). ACC/AHA/NASPE 2002 guideline for implantation of cardiac pacemakers and antiarrhythmia devices: summary article. *J Cardiovasc Electrophysiol* **13**, 1200–1.

**Indications: very general principles!**

There are only two indications for pacing (excluding pacing for heart failure):
- symptoms associated with a slow heart rate;
- a high risk of symptoms associated with a slow heart rate developing in the future.

The details of the arrhythmia are important in determining the risk of future problems and deciding how to pace the patient.

# Sinus node dysfunction

## Conduction abnormality

*Sinus node dysfunction* describes any arrhythmia that occurs because of abnormal sinus node activity—sinus bradycardia, sinus arrest (Fig. 1.19), sinoatrial block, tachyarrhythmias alternating with bradycardia or asystole. Sinus node dysfunction is associated with chronotropic incompetence (when heart rate does not increase with exercise). *Sick sinus syndrome* describes sinus node dysfunction associated with symptoms.

## Pathophysiology

Sinus node dysfunction occurs commonly with age due to degeneration of the sinus node. Other possible causes include:

- anti-arrhythmic drug therapy (e.g. digoxin, beta blocker, calcium channel antagonist, quinidine, lidocaine, procainamide);
- cardiac surgery due to direct injury to sinus node (e.g. surgery for congenital heart disease, SVC cannulation in bypass surgery);
- hypothyroidism, hypothermia;
- ischaemia;
- familial sinus node dysfunction by itself or combined with other inherited disorders (e.g. muscular dystrophy), congenital heart disease (e.g. Ebstein's, ASD), or inherited arrhythmias (e.g. ion channel disorders);
- central nervous system disease (e.g. raised ICP leading to increased parasympathetic tone).

## Indications for pacing

In symptomatic patients, rate-limiting medications should be withheld and any reversible causes (e.g. hypothyroidism) treated. If problem persists then a pacemaker should be implanted for patients:

- with symptoms that coincide with bradyarrhythmias on ambulatory monitoring (class I);
- with symptoms associated with chronotropic incompetence (class I).

A pacemaker may also be of benefit for patients:

- when symptoms are due to anti-arrhythmic drugs but the medication is needed for treatment of other problems (e.g. angina, tachycardias) (class IIa);
- when there are symptoms consistent with a bradyarrhythmia and documented sinus node dysfunction on ambulatory monitoring but symptoms were not captured on the recording (class IIa);
- with unexplained syncope and evidence of sinus node dysfunction on electrophysiological studies (class IIa).

A pacemaker can be considered for patients:

- with limited symptoms but a heart rate of < 40bpm during the daytime (class IIb).

A pacemaker is not needed if the patient is asymptomatic or recorded symptoms on ambulatory monitoring do not coincide with bradyarrhythmias captured on the same recording.

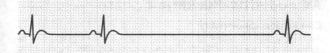

**Fig. 1.19** Example of sinus arrest.

# AV node/His–Purkinje disease

## Conduction abnormality

*AV block* describes failure of atrial electrical activity to pass from the atrium to the ventricle. Therefore, it can be secondary to dysfunction of the AV node or His bundle. Electrophysiological studies can define the block as supra-, intra-, or infra-His. There are three degrees of block:

- 1st degree AV block (Fig. 1.20)—prolongation of PR interval >200ms;
- 2nd degree AV block (type 1: Wenkebach (Fig. 1.21))—progressively lengthening PR interval then complete block of P wave (after narrow QRS complexes because block usually at level of AV node);
- 2nd degree AV block (type 2; Fig. 1.22)—fixed length PR interval before and after completely blocked P waves (often wider QRS complexes because block in His–Purkinje);
- 3rd degree AV block (Fig. 1.23)—independent P and QRS rates due to AV dissociation (often wide QRS complexes).

A fixed pattern of conducted P waves in 2nd degree block is described as 2:1, 3:1, etc. (atrial:ventricular complexes). It can be difficult to differentiate type 1 and 2 when patient is in 2:1 block as there are not enough beats to see the lengthening of the PR interval.

- The term *advanced 2nd degree AV block* can be used to describe block of two or more P waves but some conducted beats.
- *Bifascicular block* describes evidence of impaired conduction below the AV node in two of the three fascicles within the right and left bundle branches.
- *Trifascicular block,* technically, describes evidence of block in all three fascicles, such as alternating left and right bundle branch, but is also used to describe bifascicular block with any degree of AV block.

## Pathophysiology

AV node/His–Purkinje dysfunction can be congenital or acquired. Acquired block occurs due to anti-arrhythmic drugs or pathology close to the node and conducting fibres that interferes with normal function. Common causes are ischaemia, drugs (e.g. beta blockers, calcium channel antagonists, amiodarone, digoxin), or ageing of the conduction fibres with fatty infiltration and fibrosis. Other causes include:

- valvular disease (particularly calcific degeneration);
- postoperative due to direct injury or inflammation (particularly aortic valve replacement);
- AV node ablation (iatrogenic AV block);
- radiotherapy;
- infections (e.g. endocarditis of aortic valve, myocarditis, TB, syphilis, Lyme disease);
- collagen disease (e.g. scleroderma, rheumatoid arthritis, Marfan's, and ankylosing spondylitis due to aortic complications);
- infiltrative (e.g. sarcoid, amyloid, malignancy that involves the conduction system);
- neuromuscular conditions.

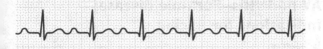

**Fig. 1.20** Example of 1st degree heart block.

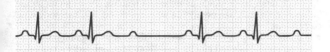

**Fig. 1.21** Example of Wenkebach 2nd degree heart block.

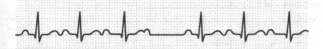

**Fig. 1.22** Example of 2nd degree heart block.

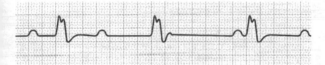

**Fig. 1.23** Example of 3rd degree heart block.

# AV node/His–Purkinje disease: indications for pacing

## Ischaemic

### Inferior myocardial infarction

AV block is common early after infarction as the right coronary artery supplies the AV node/His in 90% of the population. Block is high in the conducting system with (usually) a narrow complex escape rhythm. AV block tends to disappear as ischaemia resolves. Arrhythmias should be monitored and temporary pacing considered for haemodynamic compromise.

- If 2nd or 3rd degree AV block persists after 2 weeks this suggests permanent damage and a pacemaker should be considered (class IIa).

### Anterior myocardial infarction

AV block is ominous and implies that conduction fibres in the ventricles must be affected by a large amount of myocardial damage.

- Permanent or intermittent 2nd or 3rd degree AV block is unlikely to resolve and patients should have a pacemaker (class I).

### Bifasicular and trifasicular block after myocardial infarction

Common after infarction. Left anterior descending artery supplies both bundle branches and fascicles (although there can be circumflex and right coronary collaterals). Patients should have prolonged ECG monitoring.

- Evidence of 2nd or 3rd degree AV block suggests wider conducting system damage and a pacemaker is indicated (class I).

## Acquired

### Symptomatic 2nd and 3rd degree AV block

- If (i) there are symptoms at the time of 2nd (type 1 and type 2) or 3rd degree block, (ii) rate-limiting medications that can be stopped have been withheld, and (iii) there is not expected to be recovery from surgery or infection, patients require a permanent pacemaker (class I).
- If the patient needs a rate-limiting drug, e.g for tachycardias or angina, the medication should be combined with a pacemaker (class I).

### Asymptomatic 3rd degree heart block

In the absence of rate-limiting medications or other reversible causes—because it is very likely that the underlying problem will progress and lead to asystole or symptoms—a pacemaker is indicated if the patient is bradycardic (< 40bpm) or has pauses of > 3s (class I). A pacemaker is also probably beneficial even if not bradycardic (class IIa).

### Asymptomatic 2nd degree heart block

Site of block determines risk of higher degrees of block or asystole and therefore determines need for pacemaker.

- If at AV node (type 1) pacemaker is not indicated.
- If block below node in His–Purkinje (type 2), a pacemaker is probably beneficial (class IIa).

### 1st degree heart block

In general, a pacemaker is not required. 1st degree AV block with an extreme delay between atrial and ventricular systole, and sometimes 2nd degree AV block, can cause atrial contraction during ventricular systole. Patients develop symptoms similar to '*pacemaker syndrome*' and a pacemaker may treat the symptoms by restoring normal AV synchrony (class IIa indication).

### Bifasicular and trifasicular block

- Pacing is indicated if there is also evidence of 3rd or 2nd degree (type 2) AV block or if there is alternating bundle branch block, because these findings suggest extensive conduction system disease with a high risk of asystole (class I).
- Pacing is not indicated if there is bifasicular block with 1st degree AV block unless there are symptoms.
- Pacing can be considered in those with neuromuscular diseases and fascicular block because there is a high rate of progression of the AV conduction disease in these patients (class IIb).
- Pacing can be considered in patients with a history of syncope if there is electrophysiological evidence of a prolonged HV interval or pacing-induced infra-His block (class IIa) and other causes of syncope have been excluded.

## Congenital

### 3rd degree heart block

- If symptomatic then pacing indicated (class I).
- Risk of syncope if asymptomatic is unpredictable. Therefore these patients are often paced but, if asymptomatic with stable ventricular escape rhythm of > 50bpm, evidence for pacing is weaker.

### 2nd and 1st degree heart block

Indications are as for acquired AV block.

# Neurally mediated (vasovagal) syncope and carotid sinus hypersensitivity

## Conduction abnormality

- *Neurally mediated (vasovagal) syncope* describes a range of clinical scenarios where there is sudden failure of normal autonomic control of blood pressure and sometimes heart rate. Often episodes are provoked by factors such as posture, stress, or pain and in some patients have predictable autonomic-related triggers such as coughing, micturition, defecation, or swallowing.
- *Carotid sinus hypersensitivity* is part of this group of conditions. The neurally mediated problem is an extreme reflex response to carotid sinus massage.
- There are two components:
  - cardioinhibitory with bradycardia, asystole, or degrees of AV block due to increased parasympathetic tone;
  - vasodepressor with lowered vascular tone and hypotension due to reduced sympathetic tone.

## Pathophysiology

***Neurally mediated (vasovagal) syncope*** can present at any age. The problem is thought to be an inappropriate venous pooling in the lower body that can be worsened by standing up, hot weather, etc. This reduces the amount of blood returning to the heart, which becomes hypercontractile. There is an increased stimulation of mechanoreceptors in the heart and this is inappropriately interpreted as an increase in blood pressure, resulting in a reflex lowering of pulse rate and peripheral vascular resistance. This worsens the venous pooling and creates a cycle that leads to collapse. Situational syncope (e.g. due to micturition, coughing, etc.) is thought to occur because mechanoreceptors are also found in the bladder, rectum, oesophagus, and lungs and are triggered.

***Carotid sinus hypersensitivity*** occurs due to changes in the reflex arc involving the afferent limb from baroreceptors in the heart and carotid sinus through the glossopharyngeal and vagus nerves to brainstem and back via sympathetic and vagus nerves. It tends to occur in older people, presumably because of loss of baroreceptor function.

## Indications for pacing

Pacing is sometimes used to attenuate symptoms if there is a significant cardioinhibitory component. Medication and hydration are used for the vasodepressor component.

### Carotid sinus hypersensitivity

Medications that might be contributing and are not needed for other conditions should be stopped and then carotid sinus function assessed with massage.

- Pacing is indicated if carotid sinus massage leads to syncope and a pause of > 3s (class I) or the patient has recurrent unexplained syncope and massage causes a pause of > 3s (class IIa).

Carotid sinus hypersensitivity documented on massage but with no symptoms or history of symptoms is not an indication for pacing.

### Neurally mediated (vasovagal) syncope

Pacing should only be considered for those with significant symptoms that remain despite the patient trying to avoid precipitating behaviour or situations. If this is not possible and there are significant recurrent symptoms then the heart rate response during syncope should be recorded on ambulatory monitoring or tilt-table test. This should be used to assess the degree to which the cardioinhibitory response accounts for the symptoms.

- Pacing should be considered if there is a significant documented bradycardia associated with symptoms (class IIa). Dual chamber pacing with rate drop response is recommended (📖 p. 118).

### Is pacing useful?

Even in patients with a major cardioinhibitory component, pacing may not completely abolish symptoms but may attenuate symptoms and reduce the risk of injury. Patients should be warned that a pacemaker may not prevent syncope.

# Atrial fibrillation prevention

Pacing can be used to prevent atrial fibrillation in those with documented bradycardia-induced paroxysmal atrial fibrillation (📖 p. 126). Specific atrial preference pacing algorithms can be enabled to overdrive pace the atrium, to suppress atrial ectopics, or prevent the short–long–short sequences that may initiate arrhythmia. Atrial anti-tachycardia pacing can sometimes be used to prevent progression of atrial arrhythmias to atrial fibrillation with a programmed series of pacing stimuli that overdrive the atrium.

* Pacing is useful in the prevention of symptomatic drug-refractory recurrent atrial fibrillation in patients with coexisting sinus node dysfunction (class IIb)

# Post cardiac surgery

All types of cardiac surgery (e.g. valves, bypass surgery, congenital heart disease) can be associated with both sinus node dysfunction and AV block. This occurs due to direct injury or surgery-induced inflammation to the conducting system. Epicardial leads are often implanted at the time of surgery because of the high incidence of pacing requirement early after surgery. Abnormalities due to inflammation usually recover but if there is persistent 2nd or 3rd degree AV block after 2 or 3 weeks a permanent pacemaker will be required. Recovery is not as good after any surgery that is anatomically close to the AV node or sinus node (e.g. aortic root surgery, aortic valve replacement, or atrial septum surgery). Therefore the presence of 2nd or 3rd degree AV block a few days after surgery suggests that a permanent pacemaker will be required.

# Cardiomyopathies

In general, decisions on pacemakers in patients with cardiomyopathies should be based on the details of the arrhythmia. However, in patients with dilated cardiomyopathy, symptoms of breathlessness warrant assessment for biventricular pacing (📖 p. 282). Patients with medically refractory, symptomatic hypertrophic cardiomyopathy with significant resting or provoked left ventricular outflow obstruction can be considered for pacing (class IIb).

# Ventricular arrhythmias and pacing

Patients being considered for pacing who are at risk for ventricular arrhythmias should also be considered for an ICD (📖 p. 188) as this will provide pacing with additional defibrillator protection.

## Pause-dependent VT/long QT syndrome

- In some patients sustained ventricular arrhythmias are always reliably induced by bradycardia or pauses, with or without a prolonged QT interval, and pacing is indicated (class I).
- A similar problem can occur in patients with long QT syndrome.
- Those who are considered to be at high risk for ventricular arrhythmias based on their type of syndrome, symptoms, and ambulatory recordings can be considered for a pacemaker (class IIa)

## Pacing and ventricular arrhythmias

Patients not felt suitable for an ICD can be considered for a pacemaker combined with anti-arrhythmic drug therapy to prevent bradycardia associated with the medications.

# Syncope of unknown origin

Extensive ambulatory monitoring including insertable loop recorders (📖 p. 180) should be used to capture arrhythmias in patients with recurrent syncope to ensure an accurate diagnosis. Some patients in whom non-cardiac causes of syncope have been excluded and it has been impossible to capture an ECG recording during a syncopal episode, can be considered for a pacemaker if, clinically, it is felt that an arrhythmia is the most likely cause. However, the patient should be aware that the pacemaker may not cure the symptoms.

# Choice of pacing mode

For 95% of implants only three decisions need to be made.
1 Single or dual chamber pacing?
2 Need for rate response?
3 Need for extra functions?

Further things to be considered include the need for biventricular pacing.

### 1 Single or dual chamber (and which chambers)?

Go through these three possible steps in order.
1 Decide if there is atrial fibrillation that is not expected to resolve, be cardioverted, or treated with a pacemaker. If so, then use single lead ventricular pacing (VVI).
2 In sinus node disease, if there is no evidence of AV block and no concern that it may develop, then single lead atrial pacing can be considered (AAI).
3 If there is any evidence of AV node or His–Purkinje disease a ventricular lead is mandatory. If there are periods of sinus rhythm, dual chamber pacing (DDD) is appropriate. Exceptions to this include when the pacemaker is likely to be used infrequently for backup or there are technical problems with placing two leads, in which case single lead ventricular pacing can be used (VVI).

### 2 Need for rate response?

Go through these two possible steps in order:
1 Dual chamber pacing (DDD) and single lead atrial pacing (AAI) do not need rate response unless there is evidence of chronotropic incompetence on 24h tape or exercise.
2 Single ventricular pacing (VVI) usually requires rate response (especially when pacing-dependent). Exceptions include extreme immobility and infrequent pacing for pauses.

### 3 Need for extra functions?

All dual chamber systems (DDD) will have mode switching. Check whether the pacemaker has been prescribed for an unusual problem (e.g. atrial arrhythmias requiring anti-tachycardia pacing or neurocardiogenic syncope requiring rate drop response).

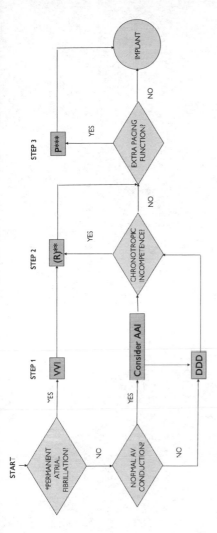

**Fig. 1.24** Choosing pacing mode. **Occasionally rate response may not be needed for VVI if pacemaker is used infrequently for backup pacing or the patient is very immobile. ***Specific pacing function will depend on the problem, e.g. anti-tachycardia pacing or rate drop response.

* If atrial fibrillation is not chronic or there is an intention to restore sinus rhythm follow the 'No' arrow.

# Permanent pacemaker implantation

# Introduction

Pacemaker therapy for bradycardia is one of the most clinically and cost-effective forms of treatment in current medicine. Heart block carries a poor prognosis and syncope is very disabling. Pacemakers may return patients to a normal life expectancy and abolish symptoms at a modest cost. However, for the patient to get the benefit of pacing the pacemaker must work properly and not become infected. Getting the pacemaker implant right is central to both of these. Adequate results are relatively easy to achieve but getting really good results needs more thought and care.

# Pre-procedure

### Operative conditions

Pacemakers are implanted foreign bodies and are prone to infection. Pacemaker infection is a disaster for the patient. At the very least sorting out a pacemaker infection is time-consuming and expensive; at worst it may be fatal. Pacemakers should therefore be implanted under optimal operating theatre conditions.

### Patient preparation

- ECG recordings demonstrating clearly the indication for pacing and used to guide mode of pacing.
- Written informed consent prior to the procedure including the following information.
  - Risks (pneumothorax, infection, tamponade, lead repositioning, pulse generator replacement).
  - Potential benefit (important when implanting CRT device or rate-drop pacemaker for vasovagal syndromes).
  - Patients should be advised that they should not drive for at least 1 week following pacemaker implant.
- Bloods.
  - FBC.
  - INR (if appropriate).
  - U & E.
- Nil by mouth 4–6h.
- Shaving implant site if required.
- Ipsilateral IV access (for sedation and venography if required).

## Antibiotic cover

Meta-analysis of randomized controlled trials of antibiotic use for pacemaker implantation supports their use but correct operating conditions and good surgical technique are probably more important. If the procedure has been prolonged or sterility suboptimal (e.g. procedure in a catheter lab) some operators give gentamicin (e.g. 80mg) to the pocket.

A typical perioperative antibiotic regimen would be:
- 1h pre-op: IV flucoxacillin 1000mg and benzylpenicillin 600mg;
- 1h post-op: IV flucoxacillin 500mg and benzylpenicillin 600mg;
- 6h post-op: oral flucoxacillin 500mg and penicillin 500mg.

For penicillin-allergic patients an alternative is vancomycin 1g over 1h started 1h pre-op.

# Implantation procedure

### Peri-procedural monitoring
This is important during implantation, especially if sedation is used. This should include:
- non-invasive BP monitoring;
- ECG;
- pulse oximetry;
- pacing system analyser (PSA).

### Scrubbing and skin draping
Optimal sterility is vital during the procedure and draping and skin preparation should be performed with the utmost care.
- The operator should wear a surgical hat and mask and then scrub for a minimum of 2min with iodine- or chlorhexidine-based scrub, before gowning-up and donning sterile gloves.
- Iodine- or chlorhexidine-based tincture should be applied liberally to the skin, then repeated, and the operating field draped including covering the patient's hair.
- Sterile self-adhesive cover (e.g. OpSite) may be applied over the dried operating field.
- Local anaesthetic (e.g. lidocaine) can then be infiltrated into the site of the skin incision and pocket.

### Left or right side?
Most implants are positioned on the non-dominant side (usually the left side as most people are right-handed). The acute angle between the right subclavian vein and SVC can sometimes cause difficulties. The only absolute reason for using the contralateral side is in patients who wish to use a shotgun (recoil could damage the skin and generator). It is now uncommon for modern systems to interfere with a golfer's swing.

A persistent left SVC (0.4% incidence) should lead to implantation on the right side unless there is an absent right SVC (rare) in which case leads can be passed via the coronary sinus to the right atrium and ventricle. This is usually discovered after the procedure has started!

### The incision and pocket
Incision site is determined mainly by venous access (most systems will be via the cephalic, subclavian or axillary vein). There are two main sites for the skin incision (Fig. 2.1):
- parallel to the clavicle (or sometimes horizontal across the anterior chest) crossing laterally to the deltopectoral groove;
- along the deltopectoral groove.

Both incisions allow access to the cephalic vein.
- The first gives better access to the subclavian vein and allows for easier fashioning of the pocket anteriorly on the chest away from the axillary skin fold.
- Incisions along the deltopectoral groove risk the pacemaker generator lying close to the edge of the chest wall increasing the risk of skin erosion.

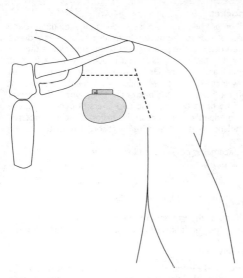

**Fig. 2.1** Positions of infraclavicular and deltopectoral incisions.

**Submuscular pocket**

Most implants will be pre-pectoral with the pocket fashioned deep to the pre-pectoral fascia, anterior to the pectoralis major muscle. All hardware should be implanted deep to the pre-pectoral fascia to minimize the risk of erosion. In very thin patients a submuscular pocket may be formed. This is more painful and may require a general anaesthetic in some patients. A shallow incision in the pectoralis major muscle allows blunt dissection through the muscle to the pectoralis minor where the pocket can be fashioned. The plane between the two layers of pectoral muscle may be difficult to identify. The pectoralis major muscle is sutured together after implant of the device using absorbable material with interrupted sutures.

Other possible pacemaker pocket positions include:
- rectus sheath (📖 p. 70);
- axilla (📖 p. 70);
- inguinal (📖 p. 70).

**Incision technique**

There are two schools of thought about the best incision technique:
- sharp dissection to the skin followed by blunt dissection to the deeper tissues;
- sharp dissection throughout.

Blunt dissection may reduce bleeding but takes longer and it may be more difficult to identify the tissue planes when closing the incision. Sharp dissection is quicker and tissue planes are easier to identify but it may be necessary to deal with more bleeding.

---

**Should you have guaranteed venous access before making the incision?**

Some operators puncture the subclavian vein to ensure a path to the right heart before making a significant incision in the patient. Being completely unable to get access to the right heart at all is very unusual but can occur. This approach also has some disadvantages. Committing to subclavian access denies the operator and the patient the advantages of using the cephalic vein. It is imperative to keep all of the hardware deep to the pre-pectoral fascia to minimize the risk of erosion. Puncturing the subclavian veins before making the incision makes it quite difficult to achieve this reliably.

# Venous access

For most purposes venous access will be either via the cephalic, sub-clavian, or axillary vein (Fig. 2.2). There are advantages and disadvantages to each technique. (See 📖 Table 2.1, p. 60 for a summary of these.)

## Cephalic vein access (Fig. 2.3)

Main advantages:
- risk of pneumothorax almost zero (may be important with underlying lung disease and 'barrel chest');
- pacing leads are within the vein during its passage between the 1st rib and clavicle hence reducing the risk of 'crush' of the lead.

The cephalic vein is located below the bright yellow fatty tissue running in the deltopectoral grove at the lateral margin of the pectoral muscles.
- Identify the vessel and dissect free with blunt dissection.
- Pass two ligatures beneath the vessel at the superior and inferior margins.
- The inferior tie can be tied off (helping to keep the operating field dry after the vein has been opened). Securing this tie in a small vein can cause it to collapse making access difficult. In this setting leaving the inferior tie loose may help.
- Keep the superior tie loose to allow passage of the lead.
- Make a small venotomy using sharp scissors.
- Using the plastic lifting hook (provided with the lead) open the venotomy and feed the pacing lead into the vein. It is often possible to pass two leads.
- After positioning the lead(s) gently tie the superior ligature to prevent leakage of blood around the lead and secure the leads to the pectoral muscle using the cuffs provided.

It may not be possible to pass a second lead due to either the vein being too small or the leads not moving freely inside the vein so preventing positioning of the leads. In this case the second lead can be placed by either the subclavian or axillary route. Although a surgical technique with a learning curve, in experienced hands two leads can be placed via the cephalic vein in most cases. A suitable cephalic vein may not be found however due to its size or presence of a network of smaller veins opposed to a single vein.

### Tips

If there is difficulty in passing the pacing wire:
- in-line traction of the ipsilateral arm may help by reducing the acute angle at the junction of the cephalic vein and axillary vein;
- make sure the superior ligature is kept loose in order not to introduce another angle or narrowing;
- gentle lifting of the vein via the inferior ligature may aid the passage of the lead;
- a guide or hydrophilic wire with a peel-away sheath may be required.

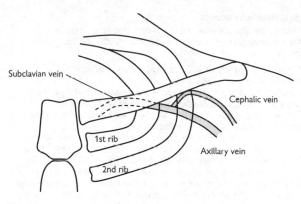

**Fig. 2.2** Anatomy of commonly used veins for pacing.

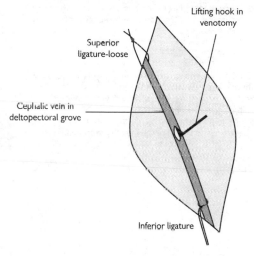

**Fig. 2.3** Cephalic vein dissection (deltopectoral incision) and position of ligatures.

### Subclavian vein access

- Main advantages are ease and speed of access in most patients.
- Main disadvantages: risk of pneumothorax (1–2%) and subclavian 'crush'.

It can be used directly or if the cephalic vein is not found or is not suitable for all leads.

- Puncture the vein under the clavicle in a relatively medial position. Using the Seldinger technique pass a peel-away sheath over the wire.
- The needle must penetrate beneath the pre-pectoral fascia so that the fascia can be closed over all the hardware.
- If puncture is straightforward it makes subsequent life easier to make two separate punctures for dual chamber systems. This reduces the friction between the two leads on positioning and reduces bleeding.
- If the puncture was not straightforward both electrodes can be placed by a single needle puncture of the subclavian vein to reduce the risks associated with multiple attempts at puncture (this requires a sheath usually 1F larger than for passing a lead alone). The guide wire of the Seldinger system is either left in the introducer sheath or replaced after the electrode has been introduced. The original sheath is removed and a second introducer sheath is passed over the original guide wire (reducing the risks associated with repeated attempts).

### Tips

- Patients kept nil by mouth may have low venous pressure so may need to be tipped head down to fill the veins.
- Contrast injection through the ipsilateral arm vein can localize the subclavian vein if access is difficult.
- Excess bleeding can be controlled by placing a purse-string suture around the electrodes as they emerge into the wound if necessary.

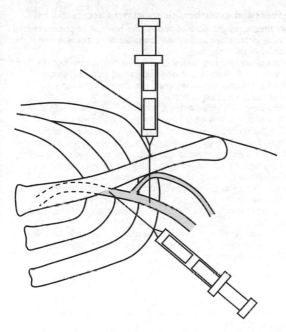

**Fig. 7.4** Extrathoracic subclavian vein puncture with tip of needle in the triangle formed by the clavicle, 1st rib, and subclavian vein. Vertical axillary vein puncture over 2nd rib after venography.

### Axillary vein and extrathoracic subclavian access (Fig. 2.4)

The main advantages are ease of access and low risk of pneumothorax and 'crush' syndrome. The axillary vein becomes the subclavian vein at the lateral border of the first rib.

- The true axillary vein may be punctured directly over the 2nd rib after venography (particularly useful when upgrading a single chamber system to a dual chamber as the puncture site will commonly be in the base of the existing pocket)
- The puncture is performed under fluoroscopy with the needle almost vertical over the 2nd rib where the venogram demonstrates the vein to pass. If the tip of the needle remains over the silhouette of the rib there is no risk of pneumothorax as the needle will stop at the rib.
- Extrathoracic subclavian vein can be punctured over the 1st rib before passing through the subclavius muscle and fascia (reducing the risk of 'crush' syndrome) without the need for a venogram.
- The needle passes at 45° to the vertical and horizontal and the tip inserted down to the 1st rib (under fluoroscopy) aiming for a triangle made by the inferior part of the clavicle, lateral margin of the 1st rib, and the vein.
- If the vein is not encountered on hitting the rib, the needle is pulled back and angled caudally. The needle can be 'walked' down the rib until the vein is encountered.

### Tip

- If an arterial puncture is inadvertently made during attempted extrathoracic subclavian access then it usually means the puncture has been made too high.
- If there is difficulty then a venogram may be performed.

**Table 2.1** Summary of advantages and disadvantages of different routes of venous access

|  | Cephalic vein | Subclavian vein | Axillary vein |
|---|---|---|---|
| Pneumothorax | < 0.1% | 1–2% | < 0.1% |
| Surgical skill | ++++ | + | + |
| 'Crush' syndrome | + | ++++ | ++ |
| X-ray | + | + | ++ |
| Ease for extraction | ++ | +++ | ++++ |
| Ease for multiple leads | + | +++ | ++++ |

# Lead implantation

### Stylets and access to the right atrium

Stylets provide stiffness to the lead, shape it, and are mouldable. They are available in different lengths (e.g. 52cm for atrial lead, 58cm for the ventricle) and stiffness. They must be kept clean and dry to ease insertion and removal from the lead. Blood in the lumen of the lead can prevent insertion of locking stylet if the lead needs removal in the future (☐ p. 313). Deflectable stylets are available where the tip of the stylet can be angled as required (useful where positioning of the lead tip is difficult).

- Usually leads pass easily to the SVC and right atrium.
- If the lead will not advance, pull back the stylet to soften the distal portion and advance again.
- If the sheath is kinked do not force the lead, but replace the guide wire and dilator and pull back the sheath a small distance and retry.
- Occasionally it is difficult to manipulate the lead through a subclavian puncture due to compression between the 1st rib and clavicle. In this case the sheath should not be removed until a final lead position is obtained. If this fails a new more lateral puncture may be required.
- When using a sheath, this can be peeled away either before or after lead positioning—if performed after lead positioning, place a stylet approximately halfway into the lead for stability and to help prevent the lead retracting during the process.

### Right ventricular lead positioning (Fig. 2.5)

- Place the RV lead first to allow for emergency RV pacing if required.
- Withdraw the stylet about 2–5cm, advance the lead to form a loop in the RA, and prolapse this across the tricuspid valve (crossing the tricuspid valve with a loop avoids inadvertently entering the coronary sinus or crossing an unrecognized ASD).
- Once across the valve unloop the lead by advancing the stylet whilst pulling the lead back.
- Conventionally the lead is placed in the RV apex near the right border of the cardiac silhouette (avoid positions near the tricuspid valve).
- If apical positions are unstable or have poor parameters change to an active lead to enable positioning in the septum or RV outflow tract.
- Leave a small loop of lead in the RA to reduce the risk of displacement during deep inspiration.
- If the lead persistently goes down the IVC the stylet will need to be curved to get a loop or to cross the tricuspid valve directly.
- If crossing the tricuspid valve is difficult, aim to get the electrode into the pulmonary artery and then replace the curved stylet with a straight one to position the electrode in the ventricle.
- It may be impossible to distinguish RV placement from coronary sinus in the AP view—LAO view will show posterior position behind the LV if the lead is in the coronary sinus and pacing will lead to RBBB pattern.
- The apex of the RV is adequate for most pacemaker patients; theoretically placement in the high septum leads a more physiological activation using the His–Purkinje system. This requires an active fixation lead.

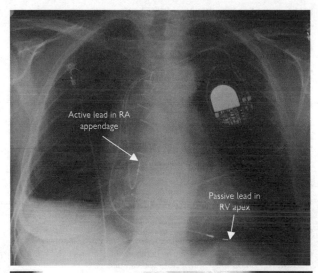

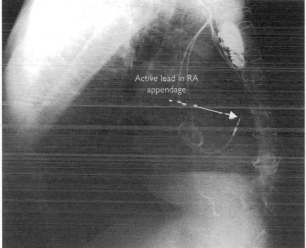

**Fig. 2.5** PA and lateral radiographs of passive lead in the RV apex and active lead in the RA appendage in patient with previous AVR. Note the anterior position of both leads on the lateral view and 'heel of the foot' appearance of the RV lead on the AP view.

## Right atrial lead positioning (Fig. 2.5)

- A preformed passive 'J' lead or active fixation 'J' or straight lead is used to position the tip in the RA appendage.
- Advance the lead down the SVC to the RA/IVC junction with a straight stylet.
- For a passive 'J', as the stylet is removed the J shape forms lifting the tip into the RA appendage. Rotation and/or retraction may be required to obtain an adequate position.
- Using an active lead a 'J' curved stylet is inserted once the tip is in the RA to position in the appendage. The screw mechanism is deployed *before* removing the stylet (an excellent test of lead stability).
- In the AP view, the tip of the lead has a 'windscreen wiper' or 'figure-of-eight' motion in patients with good appendage function. The RAO or lateral view should be used to confirm the lead tip is pointing anteriorly to the sternum.
- If poor parameters are obtained in the RA appendage, the lead should be changed to an active lead (either straight or 'J' depending on operator preference) and the lead positioned in the anterior or lateral RA.
- The atrial septum can be used if poor parameters or stability are found in the appendage (lead angled posteriorly in the LAO view).
- If the patient develops pain during deployment of the active fixation screw, reposition the lead (perforation can occur).
- Electively use active lead for patients with previous cardiac surgery.

## Securing the leads

- Using nonabsorbable material (e.g. 2/0 silk), anchor the cuffs of the leads to the pectoral muscle.
- Secure the suture to the muscle first and then around the lead cuff in two positions.
- If cephalic route used make sure the superior ligature is tied off securely but not too tightly as the suture will be directly on to the lead without a protective cuff.

# Lead implantation: electrical testing

Testing should be performed for all leads after securing the leads with stylets out of the lumen.

- Check for the presence of injury current (see box).
  - An injury current suggests good contact with endocardium.
  - No injury current is associated with higher risk of lead displacement.
- Impedance testing. Abnormal impedance may suggest insulation damage.
- Sensed P and R wave.
  - With complete heart block no sensed R wave may be seen.
  - In AF or flutter, only sensing and impedance can be measured.
- Threshold testing (Fig. 2.6).
  - Usually performed at fixed pulse width (e.g. 0.4ms), starting at high output and reducing until capture lost.
  - Threshold is lowest output that captures ventricular myocardium.
  - Usually AAI and VVI (if oversensing artefact during testing can use AOO or VOO).
- Stability testing.
  - Performed at 1.0V or twice the threshold (whichever is greater).
  - Ask patient to take a deep breath and cough.
  - Confirm no loss of capture throughout the manoeuvres.
- Pacing at maximum output (10V).
  - Exclude diaphragmatic pacing.

During atrial threshold testing the P wave may not be seen. In this case changing the lead viewed or changing to unipolar pacing may help. The sudden onset of atrial sensing on the PSA will also demonstrate loss of capture. Testing atrial capture in patients with AV nodal disease can be challenging especially when the Wenkebach point is reached. Consider the following example: resting 1st degree heart block rate the Wenkebach point is reached at 70bpm, then increasing the atrial rate to 100bpm may lead to 2:1 block, a ventricular rate of 50bpm. With loss of atrial capture ventricular rate may then increase back to 70bpm.

| Acceptable lead parameters at lead implant | | |
|---|---|---|
| | **RA lead** | **RV lead** |
| Threshold (at 0.5ms pulse width) | < 1.5V | < 1.0V |
| Sensed P/R wave | > 1.5mV | > 5mV |

If it is not possible to obtain adequate parameters the decision on what to accept depends on the underlying rhythm. For a patient with complete heart block R-wave sensing is much less important than a good threshold. Alternatively, in a patient with complete heart block with a good atrial rate then good P-wave sensing is more important than atrial threshold. Active steroid eluting leads may have a high initial threshold, which can drop significantly over a period of minutes.

### Injury current

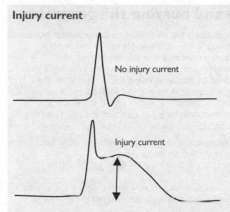

No injury current

Injury current

Presence of an injury current at time of lead placement is associated with greater lead stability. The injury current disappears over a few hours. It has been defined in studies as an increase in the duration of the atrial or ventricular intracardiac electrogram (EGM) by 50ms and an increase in ST-segment elevation of at least 5mV for ventricular leads and 1mV for atrial leads compared to baseline. Alternatively, an adequate injury current can be described as an ST-segment elevation of at least 25% of the intrinsic atrial or the ventricular electrogram amplitude. T-wave inversion can indicate partial or complete perforation.

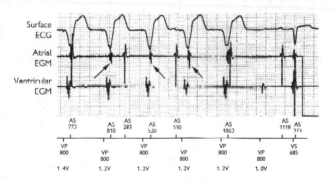

**Fig. 2.6** Ventricular threshold testing through the device showing no capture at 1.0V, i.e. threshold of 1.2V. Note the ventricular sensed event (VS) after failure to capture of the last pacing spike (VP). Atrial electrogram also demonstrates far field R-wave sensing (arrow).

## Connecting and burying the generator

Concentrate when connecting the electrodes to the generator header.
- Carelessness can result in the electrode pin not being properly through the header or in placing the pins in the wrong port.
- Check the lead identifier with your assistant before inserting it into the pacemaker header to ensure you have the correct lead.
- A pin not fully in place can work its way out with failure of pacing.
- Test the security of the connection with a tug on the electrode.
- Some operators confirm with their assistant that the pin is properly positioned in the header.

Before placing the generator in the pocket, coil any spare lead in the pocket and place the generator on top of this.
- A lead left on top of the generator can be damaged during a replacement.
- Always have a final look with fluoroscopy before closing the wound as it is possible to dislodge leads during positioning of the generator.

## Wound closure

- The wound should be closed in layers.
- Subcutaneous tissue is closed with 2/0 absorbable suture, e.g. Vicryl.
- Sutures can be interrupted or continuous.
- Skin closure is subcuticular and may be absorbable (e.g. Dexon) or non-absorbable (e.g. Prolene).
- Some operators give antibiotics (e.g. gentamicin 80mg) to the pocket.
- Surgical glue is available as an alternative to subcuticular suture.

## Post-procedure care

Patients should be advised about the following.
- Not to raise the ipsilateral arm higher than shoulder level for 6 weeks.
- The wound should be kept dry for 7 days.
- Avoid vigorous physical activities, e.g. golf, swimming, for 6 weeks.
- Non-absorbable suture should be removed at 7 days.
- Patients should be given pacemaker identity card.

## Pacemaker implantation in the anticoagulated patient

Due to risk of bleeding, patients on warfarin should be implanted with a pacemaker when the INR is below 2.0. The risks from a generator replacement are lower and local to the implant site where, as with a new implant, there is the real risk of inadvertent arterial punctures and haemothorax.

*Low risk patients on warfarin (e.g. for AF, atrial flutter)*
- Stop warfarin 5 days before implantation and check INR pre-operatively.
- Restart warfarin on the evening after implantation.

*High risk patients on warfarin (e.g. mechanical valve replacement)*
- Admit patient 3 days preoperatively and stop warfarin.
- Start IV heparin when INR < 2.0.
- Stop heparin 4h pre-procedure.
- Restart heparin 4h post-procedure and restart warfarin evening after implant.
- Alternatively, perform the implant with an INR 2–2.5 with careful use of diathermy, choice of venous access (e.g. cephalic), purse-string sutures and haemostasis.

Anecdotally, subcutaneous low molecular weight heparin is associated with a higher risk of haematoma formation.

## Management of bleeding

Bleeding is common during an implant but rarely a major problem. Generalized 'ooze' can occur without an obvious arterial bleeding source and often stops spontaneously.

*Small arterial vessels* A small pair of mosquito forceps on to the vessel and left for approximately 5min will control bleeding in most cases.

*Larger arterial vessels* Larger vessels should be clipped as above and then tied off with a length of 2/0 non-absorbable material.

*Subclavian artery puncture* If this occurs whilst attempting subclavian access direct pressure under the clavicle may be required. The operator should be aware that, if there has also been aspiration of air, there is a risk of haemo/pneumothorax.

# Other sites for pacemaker implantation

### Epicardial systems implanted in the rectus sheath

Most patients with epicardial systems will have had pacemakers implanted as neonates or very small children. The pacemaker pocket is usually fashioned in the rectus sheath deep to the rectus muscle (this form of implant is always performed by a surgeon). The original incision is midline with the rectus sheath opened behind the rectus muscle. Revision of epicardial systems can be quite physical so it is usual to perform this surgery under general anaesthesia. The cardiologists' involvement is restricted to generator changes and explants. Reopening the wound is not as easy as the first incision as scarring obscures the tissue planes but the original incision should be used to open the wound.

### Implantation in the 'axilla'

Early transvenous pacemaker systems used generators that were very large by modern standards—a similar size to an ICD. They were sometimes implanted in the 'axilla' (actually the pocket is on the lateral chest wall below the axilla). With smaller generators, made possible as lithium iodide replaced mercury zinc cells, using the 'axilla' went out of fashion. The 'axilla' pocket does have its place in children, both boys and girls.

No child likes being different so keeping the pacemaker out of sight is psychologically helpful. This position keeps the pacemaker out of the way of footballs. In girls there is no worry about asymmetric breast development from disturbance of the blood supply to the developing breast, which comes from above. As the arm is never held tightly against the side of the chest there is plenty of room for the device.

The electrode is implanted via a small incision on the front of the chest. It must be tunnelled over the edge of the pectoralis major muscle. Venous access can be either the cephalic vein or subclavian vein. A very short incision along the cephalic groove to try to find the cephalic vein can be used and, if unavailable, this incision is perfectly acceptable for subclavian puncture.

The incision for the pocket is made below the axilla. If the patient is a post-pubertal female it should be made between the top and bottom of the back-strap of the bra to minimize the amount of friction that the incision is subjected to (consider marking out a woman's bra before surgery). There is no natural tissue plane for the pocket so this must be fashioned by sharp dissection as close to the muscle layers as possible. The electrode can be pulled through from below using artery forceps or a peel-away sheath system can be used to connect the two incisions. There is usually plenty of length for the ventricular electrode but in a very tall patient a long electrode may be necessary. An atrial electrode (if required) will need to be longer than usual.

### Implantation in the groin with femoral vein access

Most pacemaker patients are elderly and may well only require one pacemaker system during their life. Patients who require pacemakers for much of their lives will require several pacemaker systems, not only generators but also electrodes. Modern lead extraction technology may be successful at maintaining venous access but, eventually, some patients will run out of access from the subclavian veins. If the SVC becomes occluded then access from above is impossible. Pacing from the groin then becomes an attractive option. Important points about femoral systems are as follows.

- A longer than normal electrode may be required and the electrode should be active rather than passive fixation.
- It is possible to implant an AV sequential system but, in a subject with this degree of pacemaker complication, keeping the pacing system as simple as possible is wise.
- The pacemaker generator needs to lie on the abdominal wall so the pocket must be above the inguinal ligament.
- The incision should be above the groin crease so it is not affected by flexing the hip.
- There is a more direct route from the right femoral vein to the heart compared to the left (the right femoral vein crosses behind the femoral artery, usually between the groin crease and the inguinal ligament, so the venous puncture needs to be below the incision).
- To prevent the generator migrating down into the groin the pacemaker pocket should be closed with insoluble suture material either continuous or interrupted.

The tissues and skin can be closed in the usual way.

### Supraclavicular vein access

The supraclavicular approach is useful:
- when it is not possible to obtain access via the axillary, cephalic, or infraclavicular subclavian vein;
- for a tunnelled temporary pacing system following extraction for infection whilst awaiting a new permanent system (📖 p. 313).

# Special considerations in the young

Pacing patients for the whole of their life will certainly result in problems. The decision to recommend pacemaker therapy in the very young is not taken without a great deal of care but, having done so, plans need to be in place from the beginning to maximize the longevity of each access site so that the patient doesn't run out of sites.

For this reason it is helpful if adult pacemaker specialists are involved in pacing children as adult cardiologists see and have to deal with the consequences of paediatric cardiologists' decisions.

General principles for pacing the younger patient are as follows.
- Therapy should be the simplest that will achieve the aim.
- If at all possible transvenous pacing should be avoided before the age of 2 years.
- Pacing should be delayed for as long as possible after that age.
- The generator should be out of sight and out of harm's way from footballs, etc.
- Minimize the consequences of growth.

## Pacing children in the neonatal period

A pacemaker in a neonate should be epicardial. Epicardial pacemakers are usually reliable for a few years and can occasionally get the individual into full adult life before any transvenous access is necessary. If venous access can be delayed until the patient is 20 years of age there is a very good chance of getting through the entire life without substantial complications. The further the epicardial system can be kept working in childhood the better, as the long-term benefits of allowing the child to grow as much as possible before going transvenous mount up rapidly.

Every attempt possible should be made to keep an epicardial system going, including repair of fractured epicardial electrodes, in order to avoid the need for transvenous access for years.

Children are close to half their adult height at the age of 2 years. Delaying the use of the transvenous system until at least this age substantially reduces the consequences of growth.

## Pacing larger children and young adults

Pacemaker implantation in children is usually under general anaesthetic.
- The cephalic vein should be used if it is available to reduce the chances of occlusion of the subclavian vein.
- An active fixation electrode should be used as these are easier to extract.
- New lumenless 4F pacing leads are available and may be considered. The downside of these is the lack of a lumen when it comes to lead extraction (💷 p. 318).
- Leave ample slack in the electrode and, if the child has a lot of growing to do, a complete loop should be left in the right atrium.
- Consider placing the generator in the axilla to avoid the impact of a pre-pectoral device in children.

## Single or dual chamber pacing in children?

The indication for pacing is to prevent sudden death and syncope. This will be reliably achieved by VVI(R) pacing (including rate responsiveness). The temptation to change the pacemaker system to an AV sequential device should be resisted. Changing from VVI to DDD pacemaker prescription should not necessarily be regarded as an 'upgrade'.

# Pulse generator replacement

# General principles

As with any procedure the indication for a pulse generator replacement should be confirmed prior to starting and the device fully assessed. It is important to assess the leads as the presence of a lead defect may convert a 'simple box change' into a revision with an additional lead or consideration of a lead extraction. As well as the lead parameters, before proceeding it is important to confirm the compatibility of lead pins with the new pulse generator, especially with older systems of the pre IS-1 era. Adapters are available for older leads.

The underlying rhythm and the configuration of the leads (unipolar or bipolar) should be known before the procedure. In pacemaker-dependent patients, temporary pacing should be considered and, for patients with no underlying rhythm or who are unable to tolerate a slow ventricular escape, it is necessary. Some pacemakers used for the treatment of atrial arrhythmias need bipolar leads. If one is to be implanted the lead type already in place needs to be known.

The risk of infection or wound revision is higher for a generator replacement than for a new system and attention to detail is important.

# Patient preparation

- Obtain consent for the implantation of a new lead as well as a pulse generator replacement in case at testing a lead defect is discovered. There is also the potential for damage to old leads during removal of the old generator.
- Antibiotics (📖 p. 51) are given routinely pre- and peri-procedure as for a new implant. This is supported by retrospective data.
- If required insert temporary pacing wire (📖 p. 168) via femoral vein (this should be performed before preparing the permanent pacemaker site and the operator should rescrub before proceeding).
- Skin preparation and local anaesthesia infiltration are as for a new implant (📖 p. 52).

## Pulse generator replacement

# Pulse generator replacement

## Removal of pulse generator

- For a pulse generator replacement alone, make the incision over the generator, usually below the position of previous implantation scar (reducing the risk of damage to the existing leads, which should be below, superior, or lateral to the generator).
- For cosmetic reasons the incision may be made at the site of the previous incision, although this increases the risk of damage to the leads.
- Dissect down to the capsule around the generator using blunt dissection. The capsule may be a thin translucent layer or have significant fibrosis and some calcification, especially in the elderly.
- Make a small incision in the capsule with a scalpel on to the generator having confirmed that no lead is present under the point of incision.
- Extend the incision by careful use of scissors until the box can be explanted.
- Fibrosis around the leads as they enter the header may occur and require dissection so that sufficient lead can be freed to detach the old generator and connect the new one. In some cases with extensive fibrosis, diathermy may be required.
- Unscrew the set screws and detach the generator.

## Check of existing leads

- Check all leads through the PSA even if interrogation of the device before removal has demonstrated normal lead function.
- Check the threshold and impedance as damage to lead insulation may have occurred during removal of the generator.

## New generator implantation

- The pocket for the new generator will often need to be expanded medially and/or inferiorly to accommodate the new generator.
- Avoid extending the pocket laterally as this may lead to migration of the device towards the axilla.
- Failure to have a large enough pocket may lead to difficulty in closing the wound adequately and increase the risk of infection and later erosion.

## Undoing the set screws

The set screws are undone using a hexagonal screwdriver or wrench. Although a simple procedure it is important that this is performed carefully. Before rotating the screwdriver or wrench make sure that it is fully inserted into the head of the set screw. Failure to do so can result in breaking the tip of the wrench off completely, making it impossible to remove the lead from the device. This may make it necessary to cut the lead and to implant a new lead (it may be possible to repair a unipolar lead).

# Downgrading from dual chamber to single chamber

It is quite common for patients to reach generator replacement with an existing dual chamber system yet require only single chamber pacing (usually patients developing permanent atrial fibrillation having previously been in sinus rhythm). Therefore a single chamber pulse generator may be implanted and the atrial lead not used. In case lead extraction is required in the future, blood must be prevented from entering the lumen of the lead. Two options are available.

- Cover the lead pin with a dedicated silicone cap (Fig. 3.1) placing a ligature around it to keep it in place.
- Cut the lead, pull the conducting inner core from within the insulation, and cut further down the lead to leave the insulation longer than the core. Place a ligature around the area of insulation only to seal it. (Fig. 3.2).

For active fixation leads, the pin should be capped so that if extraction is required in the future the screw mechanism can be withdrawn. Having covered the lumen of the lead, the lead should be sutured to the base of the pocket to prevent migration of the lead.

# Addition of a new lead and generator replacement

- A new lead may be required due to an upgrade of a single to a dual chamber system or due to failure of an existing lead. In the latter case a careful decision is required whether to leave the existing lead in place or to extract it.
- If the addition of a new lead has been planned and existing leads have been in place for a long time then an ipsilateral venogram may be performed to assess patency of the venous system.
- The incision site depends on the access to be used—a standard generator replacement incision can often be made and, following a venogram, an axillary vein puncture over the second rib may be made (📖 p. 58).
- If the generator is quite inferior then two incisions may be necessary and the new lead tunnelled from the access point to the pocket.

# Pocket revision

The time of generation replacement is an ideal opportunity for any revision of the pocket, e.g. with a generator that has migrated towards the axilla or subpectoral placement for patients with weight loss and little subcutaneous tissue and potential erosion.

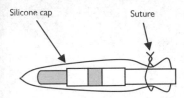

**Fig. 3.1** Silicone cap sealing the lead core.

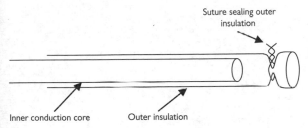

**Fig. 3.2** Sealing the lead insulation. The inner core is cut shorter than the outer insulation, and a non-absorbable suture used to seal it to prevent ingress of blood into the lumen of the lead.

# Pacemaker complications

# Introduction

Although pacemaker implantation is a relatively simple technique there are significant complications, which can be divided broadly into the time of presentation: peri-procedural; intermediate; and late.

# Peri-procedural complications

These complications become apparent during the procedure or in the immediate perioperative period.

### Failed venous access

In some patients during the procedure it may not be possible to access the heart via the cephalic or subclavian veins, especially if leads are already in place (📖 p. 56). Alternative sites should be considered and expert help sought.

### Pneumothorax and haemothorax

Pneumothorax occurs following puncture of the pleural space while obtaining venous access (Fig. 4.1). The risk of pneumothorax from a blind subclavian puncture is 1–1.5% and with cephalic or axillary vein approach is almost zero. Haemothorax is less common and can occur from damage to the subclavian artery or vein—although usually benign it can be life-threatening.

- Sudden onset of shortness of breath, change in blood pressure, or oxygen desaturation should alert the operator to the possibility.
- Fluoroscopy may be diagnostic but image quality is poor compared to a CXR.
- Often a pneumothorax will be small, asymptomatic, and picked up on the post-procedure CXR.
- Management is along standard guidelines.
- A chest drain kit should be readily available in the pacing theatre.

### Air embolus

This can occur with any access route when a sheath is used and can be avoided by instructing the patient to avoid taking deep inspirations, using the smallest sheath that is required, and occluding the sheath when appropriate.

- Small volumes of air can embolize to the right heart and are usually well tolerated. Large volumes may lead to chest pain, hypotension, hypoxaemia, and cardiac arrest.
- Treatment is with high flow oxygen and, rarely, inotropic support may be required.

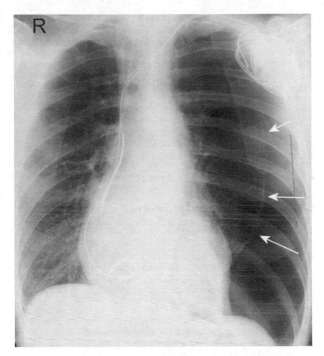

**Fig. 4.1** Left-sided pneumothorax (arrowed) following implantation of a biventricular ICD.

### Important points following failed venous access

- Having failed to obtain subclavian or axillary access on one side, attempts to obtain access on the opposite side are not recommended due to the potential for the development of bilateral pneumothoraces.
- Venography may be performed prior to a second procedure to confirm access.

### Cardiac perforation and tamponade (Figs 4.2 and 4.3)

This can occur when a lead is passed across the atrial or ventricular septum into another cardiac chamber or into the pericardial space. Sub-clinical right ventricular perforation is probably more common than reported. Overall risk of tamponade during pacing procedures is approximately 0.2%. Risk factors for perforation include increasing age, female sex, steroid use. Soft stylets should be used wherever possible to reduce risk.

- Early signs of tamponade are tachycardia and progressive hypotension. However, a sinus tachycardia may not occur in chronotropically incompetent patients.
- T-wave inversion on the intracardiac EGM may indicate perforation.
- Echocardiography allows rapid diagnosis.
- Treatment of the effusion should be along standard guidelines.
- A pericardiocentesis kit should always be available in the pacing theatre.

### Left ventricular (LV) lead placement

Inadvertent placement of a lead in the LV may occur through an ASD/PFO or VSD. It is also possible to place the lead in a coronary vein via the coronary sinus (CS).

- It may be impossible to distinguish placement in the LV or RV on AP fluoroscopy but lateral views will demonstrate the posterior position of the lead.
- A 12 lead ECG will demonstrate RBBB morphology with LV pacing.
- A lead in the LV should be removed as soon as possible due to the risk of thromboembolism.

### Poor stability or inadequate threshold/sensing

If there is difficulty in obtaining adequate sensing and pacing parameters or poor stability with a passive lead, then it may be necessary to change to an active lead (📖 pp. 12–13) and consider alternative pacing sites (e.g. lateral right atrium, right ventricular septum).

- Occasionally there is difficulty in obtaining a good position in the RV in patients with severe tricuspid regurgitation and, if an active lead can not be positioned, then it may be necessary to use a CS catheter to position the lead (📖 p. 294).
- New 4F leads are now available using a sheath similar to a CS sheath.

### Subclavian artery puncture

This can occur during attempted blind puncture of the subclavian.

- In most cases the presence of pulsatile flow will raise suspicions. However, if venous pressure is high it can be difficult to differentiate between arterial and venous access.
- Passing the guide wire into the IVC below the diaphragm confirms a venous puncture. Check with fluoroscopy before inserting the sheath.
- In most cases simple pressure will prevent complications although haemothorax (📖 p. 84) can occur.

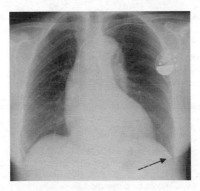

**Fig. 4.2** Perforation of the right ventricular apex with the tip of a passive lead (arrowed) lateral to cardiac silhouette.

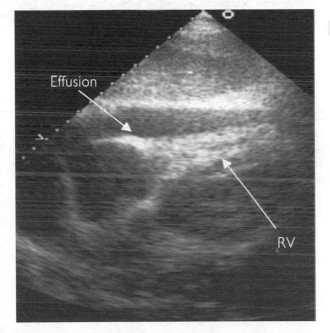

**Fig. 4.3** Subcostal view demonstrating tamponade with large pericardial effusion and collapse of the RV.

# Intermediate complications

These become apparent some hours/days after the procedure.

## Haematoma

- Small haematomas at the site of implant may occur and should be managed conservatively as re-opening the pocket increases the risk of infection.
- A pressure dressing can be applied if a haematoma is suspected or developing.
- If at all possible avoid re-opening the wound as this may introduce infection.
- Unless absolutely necessary, withhold anticoagulants for a few days.
- If there is continued bleeding, massive haematoma, breakdown of the skin sutures and/or major discomfort, evacuation and inspection for the bleeding site should be performed.

## Micro/macrodislodgement of lead tip

- *Macrodislodgement* refers to movement of the tip of the pacing wire that is visible radiographically. This may require lead repositioning and should be performed as soon as possible.
- *Microdislodgement* refers to movement of the tip that is not visible radiographically but alters either the sensing or pacing abilities of the lead. The need for lead revision depends on the lead parameters.

# Late complications

Late complications occur anywhere between a few days and a few years after implantation.

### 'Twiddler's syndrome'

Patients can rotate the device in the pocket dragging a lead out of position (Fig. 4.4).
- Leads may need repositioning and the generator may be placed subpectorally to reduce the risk of recurrence.

### Venous thrombosis

Asymptomatic thrombosis in the vessel related to the leads is quite common. Silent vessel occlusion occurs in 10–15% of patients. It is more common with multiple leads. Therefore, in younger patients, if a new lead is required, it may be advisable to extract the old lead.
- Symptomatic thrombosis of the axillary or subclavian system leads to venous engorgement and pain in the ipsilateral limb. Pulmonary embolism may occur but is very rare.
- Diagnosis is with venography.
- Management includes elevation, anticoagulation, and occasionally thrombolysis.
- SVC obstruction can occur but is rare and is thought to be related to thrombus and fibrosis.
- Management can be difficult and may involve endovascular reconstruction, stenting, and lead extraction.

### Infection, erosion, and wound problems

Infection can occur directly related to a pacemaker procedure but also from unrelated procedures that may result in bacteraemia (e.g. skin infections/trauma) and subsequent colonization of the pacing system. Infection is more common following box change compared to new system implants (probably related to poor wound closure).
- Threatened erosion with thin covering tissue, bruising of the skin, and inflammation can occur following weight loss or a poorly fashioned pocket and this can be treated by box repositioning (may require submuscular pocket) before erosion occurs.
- Erosion describes the exposure of the system through the skin. There is a significant risk of infection and this requires extraction.
- Infected pacemakers invariably require system (generator and lead) extraction (🕮 p. 313).
- 'Winged' lead-securing cuffs are used to prevent migration of the sheath into veins. If these cuffs rotate the 'wings' can push up towards the skin and cause pain and/or threatened erosion. The wings can be cut free from the main body of the cuff.

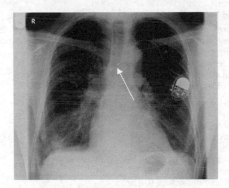

**Fig. 4.4** 'Twiddler's syndrome' with retraction of the ventricular lead (arrow) back into the SVC with the excess lead coiled in the pocket

## Lead and insulation fracture

Lead failures may occur due to manufacturing defect, but more commonly due to extrinsic forces applied to the lead. These commonly occur at three sites:
- suture sleeve, due to excessively tight suture;
- between clavicle and 1st rib;
- friction of lead with other lead or box.

Lead insulation fractures may present as:
- distortion of the insulation on CXR;
- pectoral stimulation;
- 'unipolarization' of a bipolar lead with an increased pacing spike amplitude similar to that of a unipolar lead;
- reduced amplitude of pacing spike with a unipolar lead;
- increased capture threshold (📖 p. 134);
- reduced lead impedance (📖 p. 136).

Conduction fractures can lead to a complete open circuit with no electrical continuity (extremely high impedance). A similar situation can occur with failure to secure the set screw. This may present as:
- failure to pace with no pacing spike;
- massively elevated lead impedance.

Incomplete conduction fractures may present as:
- reduced amplitude of pacing spikes;
- loss of capture;
- failure to pace due to oversensing;
- intermittent problems may lead to transient changes in lead impedance outside of the normal range;
- oversensing and undersensing will be discussed later in detail (📖 pp. 138–147).

## Exit block

Inflammation at the electrode–myocardial interface can be severe leading to fibrosis and exit block (📖 p. 136).
- Becomes apparent by a steady but gradually increasing threshold.
- The use of steroid eluting electrode tips has reduced the frequency of exit block (incidence < 5%).
- Anecdotally, oral steroids have been used.
- A new lead is invariably needed if pacing parameters are unacceptable, rather then repositioning the old lead (steroid will have been depleted).

## Pacemaker syndrome

This is not a true complication of the procedure but is usually caused by VVI pacing in people with sinus rhythm and dissociated atrial contraction. The lack of synchrony between atrial and ventricles leads to intermittent atrial contraction i.e. with closed AV valves. Alternatively ventricular pacing may activate the atria if retrograde AV node conduction is present. Symptoms include fatigue, dizziness, neck pulsation, breathlessness, and postural hypotension. Upgrading to a dual chamber device restores AV synchrony and usually abolishes symptoms.

# Pacemaker programming and device interrogation

# Lower rate interval

The *lower rate interval* (LRI) determines the minimum rate (*lower rate limit,* LRL) at which chambers are paced (atrial paced (AP) or ventricular paced (VP)) and therefore determines the *bradycardia rate*. It is the maximum time allowed between one sensed or paced beat and the next. If a sensed (atrial sensed (AS) or ventricular sensed (VS)) event is not detected during that time interval, the chamber will be paced. It may be measured in milliseconds or beats per minute.

- In *single chamber modes* (AAI or VVI) the atrial or ventricular rate should not fall below the programmed bradycardia rate (□ p. 22).
- In *dual chamber modes* (DDD, DDI) neither the atrial nor the ventricular rate should fall below the *bradycardia rate* (□ p. 24).
- In *VDD mode* the atrial rate may fall below the LRL as there is no atrial pacing, but the ventricular rate will not (□ p. 24).
- In *dual chamber tracking modes*, i.e. DDD, the LRI may be atrial-based or ventricular-based.
  - With an *atrial-based* LRI, the minimum atrial rate (AS–AP or AP–AP) is the constant and equals the programmed lower rate limit, regardless of subsequent AV conduction (AVI) and atrial escape interval (VP–AP or VS–AP). V–V times may be equal to, slightly shorter than, or slightly longer than the LRL.
  - With a *ventricular-based* LRI, the atrial escape interval AEI (VP–AP or VS–AP) is the constant. The atrial escape interval equals LRI – AVI. The A–A times and the V–V times may be equal to, slightly shorter than, or slightly longer than the LRL.

If a paced chamber's rate is noted to have fallen below the LRL, there may be a problem with sensing or stimulation.

## Choosing a lower rate limit

The choice of *lower rate limit* is determined by the pacing indication and the presence of intermittent or constant bradycardia or heart block. The goal is to achieve a physiological heart rate, avoid bradycardia symptoms, and minimize pacing (to conserve battery life and avoid potentially detrimental RV pacing). Remember that the LRL will normally also apply at night, when the patient is asleep and the natural, physiological heart rate is normally slow. Suggestions for specific situations are given in the box opposite.

## Related programming features

*Hysteresis* can minimize ventricular pacing by allowing the intrinsic rate to drop very low before pacing starts at a faster rate (□ p. 116).

*Sleep function* The sleep function can lower the LRL during sleep periods to avoid heartbeat awareness (□ p. 120).

## Programming LRL in specific conditions

*Infrequent pauses* Pacing is only rarely required and a LRL of 40–50bpm may be suitable to prevent symptoms while avoiding unnecessary pacing for the majority of time.

*Chronic, persistent bradycardia* Constant pacing is usually required and the LRL is often set to a 'physiological' 60bpm.

*Relative bradycardia* For conditions in which a relative bradycardia may be detrimental (long-QT syndrome, bradycardia-induced arrhythmias such as atrial fibrillation or VT), a LRL of 70–80bpm may be chosen. Faster rates may increase cardiac output in certain disease conditions and usually only with AV synchrony.

*Detrimental fast heart rates* For conditions in which a faster rate may be detrimental (e.g. angina) a slower lower rate limit of 50–60bpm may be appropriate, particularly in VVI pacing mode.

*VVI* If the underlying rhythm is sinus rhythm with intact AV conduction and the pacing mode is VVI, pacing will result in AV dissociation and possibly pacemaker syndrome. The slowest LRL that abolishes brady-cardia symptoms is therefore required to encourage normal AV conduction. In chronic atrial fibrillation a resting rate of 60–70bpm may be more appropriate.

## Rate smoothing

Rate smoothing is designed to avoid marked changes in cycle length when pacing rate increases from LRL or decreases from the upper rate limit (URL). A rate-smoothing algorithm introduces a limit on the percentage change in paced ventricular intervals, e.g. 3%, 6%, 9%, or 12% of the preceding R–R interval. This applies throughout the entire range of atrial sensing (from LRI to URI). Although changes in ventricular rate are relatively smooth, this may result in the transient loss of AV synchrony until the ventricle 'catches up' with the atrium.

# Upper rate interval

The *upper rate limit* (URL) determines the fastest rate at which a pacemaker will pace a chamber and is defined by *upper rate interval* (URI).

- Single chamber pacing modes with inhibition only, and non-tracking dual chamber modes (AAI, VVI, DVI, and DDI) only have URLs if they have rate response (AAIR, VVIR, VDIR, and DDIR) programmed.
- Dual chamber pacing modes with triggering (tracking modes: DDD or VDD) have a URL that is the maximum rate at which the ventricle can be paced in response to atrial sensed or paced events and maintain 1:1 AV conduction. In this situation it is also called the *maximum tracking rate* (MTR). (See Fig. 5.1.)

## Exceeding the upper rate limit

- If the intrinsic atrial rate exceeds the URL (e.g. during sinus tachycardia or atrial fibrillation) and there is intrinsic AV conduction, the ventricular rate may exceed the URL and ventricular pacing will be inhibited.
- If the intrinsic atrial rate exceeds the URL and there is no intrinsic AV conduction (e.g. complete heart block) then a Wenckebach or 2:1 AV response occurs.

## Choosing the upper rate limit

Choose a URL that is appropriate for the level of activity that the patient is likely to undertake, as far as the AV delay and post-ventricular atrial refractory period (PVARP) will allow.

- Young, active patients may require URLs of 150bpm.
- Angina patients may need URLs ≤ 110 bpm to avoid chest pain.

---

### Upper rate limit and total atrial refractory period

- The *upper rate interval* cannot be shorter than the *total atrial refractory period* (TARP, which equals AVI + PVARP). The TARP represents the total time during which the atrial channel ignores any sensed events and therefore cannot act on them.
- With atrial cycle lengths between the URI and TARP a Wenckebach response occurs (Fig. 5.2(a)). In this scenario, the AVI is completed before the URI time period from the previous ventricular beat has been reached. The pacemaker extends the AVI until the URI is reached, and then paces the ventricle.
- If the *sensed* atrial cycle length is shorter than the TARP, a fixed, 2:1 response will occur (Fig. 5.2(b)).
- Making sure the TARP is shorter than the URI avoids a sudden drop in ventricular rate following an abrupt onset of 2:1 block when the URI is exceeded. This can be achieved by:
  - programming a short sensed AV interval;
  - having a dynamic sensed AV interval that shortens as the atrial rate increases (📖 p. 100);
  - programming a shorter PVARP;
  - having a dynamic PVARP that shortens as the atrial rate increases.

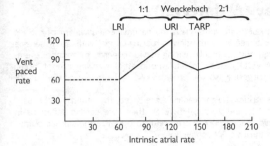

**Fig. 5.1** Upper rate limit and atrial tracking. Effect of increasing sensed atrial rate on the paced ventricular rate in DDD tracking mode. There is a 1:1 response between the LRL of 60bpm and URL of 120bpm. Above the URI, AV Wenckebach occurs. When the TARP (AVI + PVARP) is exceeded, a 2:1 response occurs.

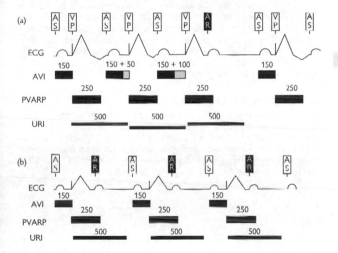

**Fig. 5.2** AS = atrial sensed; AR = atrial refractory; VS = ventricular sensed; VP = ventricular paced. (a) Upper rate response: AV Wenckebach. Sensed atrial rate of 130bpm (450ms) is above URL of 120bpm (500ms). Each AVI is extended by an additional 50ms to stop the URI from being exceeded. After three sensed events, the extension of the AVI causes the 4th sensed event to fall in the PVARP so it is ignored. (b) Upper rate response: 2:1. Atrial rate is now 170bpm (350 ms). As the cycle length is shorter than the TARP (400ms) alternate atrial events fall within the PVARP and are ignored. The paced ventricular rate is therefore half the atrial rate.

# AV delay (AV interval)

The *atrioventricular interval* (AVI) is the pacemaker equivalent of the PR interval. It is a requirement for any pacing mode with atrial sensing (and/or pacing) and ventricular pacing that is triggered by an atrial event, i.e. DDD or VDD modes. In DDI mode atrial tracking cannot occur (there is no triggering) so the programmed AVI represents the AP–VP interval.

If both the atrium and the ventricle are paced, the optimal AVI is usually between 125 and 200ms. However, there are certain situations in which dynamic changes in AVI are useful to optimize the cardiac output or encourage intrinsic AV conduction.

## Difference between sensed and paced AV delays (Fig. 5.3)

Paced and sensed AV delays are usually different. This is because atrial activity is sensed when activation is already underway (usually from the sinus node), the P wave has already begun, and activation is already part of the way to the AV junction. If atrial activation is paced, the pacing site is the earliest part of the atrium to be activated, the P wave hasn't begun, and it will take longer for activation to reach the AV junction. Therefore the *sensed AVI* is often programmed 20–50ms shorter than the *paced AVI*. A shorter *sensed AVI* also means a shorter TARP which allows a faster URL in tracking modes and avoids sudden onset of 2:1 block at high atrial rates.

## Rate-adaptive AVI (Fig. 5.4)

The normal physiological PR interval is 120–200ms. In normal subjects the PR interval shortens by 20–50ms with exercise. *Rate-adaptive AVI* (dynamic AV delay) allows the pacemaker AVI (AS–VP with an increase in intrinsic rate, AP–VP with increased sensor activity) to shorten, mimicking exercise physiology and allowing a shorter TARP and a faster URL.

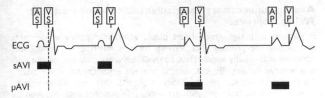

**Fig. 5.3** Sensed and paced AVIs. The sensed AV interval (sAVI) is programmed at 150ms, whereas the paced AVI (pAVI) is programmed at 200ms.

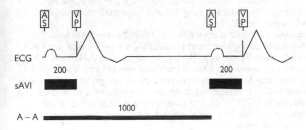

**Fig. 5.4** Rate-adaptive AVI. The faster the atrial rate, the shorter the AV interval, within a programmable range.

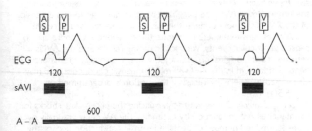

### Avoiding unnecessary ventricular pacing—when is a long AVI appropriate?

In patients with high grade heart block, ventricular pacing is inevitable and usually the primary goal. Where there is intrinsic AV conduction, however, it is usually appropriate to minimize ventricular pacing, not only to conserve battery life but also to prevent potential harm. RV pacing results in ventricular dyssynchrony in hearts that may otherwise be activated in a normal, synchronous fashion. In patients with impaired LV systolic function, this dyssynchrony may reduce cardiac output, impair exercise capacity, and worsen heart failure.

Avoidance of unnecessary RV pacing may be achieved by the following.

- Programming an AVI longer than the intrinsic PR interval (e.g. 200–280ms). This may not be possible if there is significant 1st degree heart block. A long AVI also lowers the maximum programmable URL.
- *Managed ventricular pacing algorithm*. MVP (Medtronic) is an atrial-based pacing mode that provides the safety of a dual chamber backup mode if necessary. The pacemaker starts in AAI mode. If there are two successive atrial sensed or paced events without an intrinsic ventricular sensed event in between there is a single backup ventricular paced beat. If intrinsic conduction does not return the pacemaker switches to DDD mode. The pacemaker will subsequently check again for intrinsic AV conduction and, if it has returned, switch back to AAI mode.
- *AV delay hysteresis*. Each company has a variation of the same theme. In some, AV delay hysteresis is initiated after a consecutive number of paced ventricular beats (a 'look–see'). In others, AV delay hysteresis occurs only after a sensed ventricular event occurs during the programmed AVI. The pacemaker applies a programmed extension of the AVI in the next cycle. If there is continued ventricular sensing, the AVI remains extended. If, despite the extended AVI, there are no sensed ventricular events, ventricular pacing results and the AVI is returned to the original programmed value. Ventricular premature beats that fall within the AVI will mimic intrinsic conduction and may also initiate AV delay hysteresis if this option is programmed on (Fig. 5.5(a), (b)).
- *AV delay scanning*. During ventricular pacing the pacemaker checks for spontaneous AV conduction by extending the AV delay gradually over a predetermined number of beats. If intrinsic conduction occurs, the AVI remains at the new, extended value.

### When is a short AVI appropriate?

- Some patients with hypertrophic obstructive cardiomyopathy and a high left ventricular outflow tract gradient may have their gradient reduced by RV apical pacing.
- CRT pacing usually requires a shorter AV delay (80–120ms) to ensure 100% ventricular pacing and also to optimize cardiac output (📖 p. 306).
- Short AVIs lead to shorter TARPs and facilitate shorter URIs and a more physiological response to faster atrial rates during exercise.

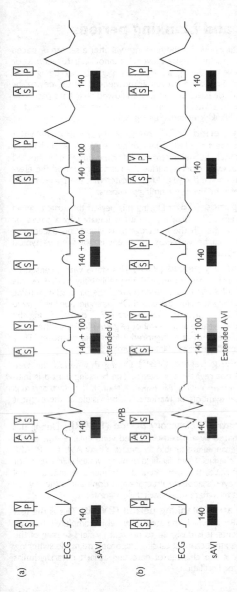

**Fig. 5.5** (a) AV delay hysteresis. The programmed sAVI is 140ms. A sensed ventricular event due to intrinsic conduction that took only 130ms initiates an immediate prolongation of the AVI by 100ms to look for any further evidence of intrinsic AV conduction. This happens with the next beat, although intrinsic conduction takes longer (210ms). In the following beat, there is no sensed ventricular activity after 240ms so ventricular pacing occurs, restoring the sAVI to the nominal value of 140ms. (b) AV delay hysteresis. In this example, a patient with complete heart block has a programmed sAV of 140ms. A premature ventricular beat occurs 60ms after a sensed P wave (i.e. within the sAVI), which initiates the AV search. The sAVI is extended by 100ms to 240ms; however, as there is complete heart block ventricular pacing is still required after 240ms and the sAVI returns to the nominal value for subsequent beats.

# Refractory and blanking periods

A pacemaker *refractory period* is the time interval after a sensed or paced event during which further sensed events cannot initiate actions or counters. Sensed events during a refractory period may be ignored completely (*blanked*) and are not even acknowledged by the device, or they may be ignored for basic functions but allowed to initiate particular algorithms (e.g. mode switching with high atrial rates). All *refractory periods* begin with a *blanking period*. (See Fig. 5.6.)

**Atrial refractory period (ARP)** An atrial signal falling within this time period will not affect the LRI or initiate a new AVI. In dual chamber pacing modes, the atrial channel is refractory for the duration of the AVI (ARP = AVI). If atrial events occur during the refractory period the electrogram is visible and a symbol (e.g. AR) indicates that the pacemaker is aware but has ignored the event for timing purposes.

**Atrial blanking period (ABP)** During this period the atrial channel will not register events. The blanking period is initiated by a paced or sensed atrial event. Although the electrogram is visible, no pacemaker symbols or markers will be visible as the event is not seen. A typical value would be 30–50ms.

**Ventricular refractory period (VRP)** This starts with a sensed or paced ventricular event and is a period during which any further events have no effect on the LRI. VRPs are used to avoid the pacemaker sensing its own ventricular stimulus, the paced QRS complex, or the T wave that follows the QRS complex. If a ventricular event occurs during the VRP the electrogram is visible and a symbol (e.g. VR) indicates the pacemaker is aware of the event but has ignored it for timing purposes. They are usually programmed between 200 and 300ms.

**Ventricular blanking period (VBP)** During this period the ventricular channel will not register any events. The blanking period is initiated by a paced or sensed ventricular event. Although the electrogram is visible, no pacemaker symbols or markers will be visible as the event is not seen.

**Post-ventricular atrial refractory period (PVARP)** During this period, which is initiated by a paced or sensed ventricular event, events sensed in the atrial channel are unable to initiate a new AVI. The PVARP prevents the atrial channel from far-field sensing ventricular events or sensing retrograde P waves that may occur due to intact ventricular–atrial conduction. Sensed events appear refractory and don't affect the AVI or LRI but may be used to initiate mode-switching algorithms.

**Post-ventricular atrial blanking period (PVAB)** This is the first portion of the PVARP in which the atrial channel is completely blanked from any sensed events. It is designed to prevent far-field sensing of the QRS complex by the atrial channel causing inappropriate mode switching. A long PVAB reduces the chances of detecting atrial tachyarrhythmias such as atrial flutter or fibrillation.

**Post-atrial ventricular blanking (PAVB)** This is a short interval (< 60ms) that switches off sensing in the ventricular channel immediately after atrial pacing (but not sensing). It prevents the ventricular channel from inappropriately sensing the atrial pacing stimulus (more likely to happen with unipolar systems). If the PAVB period is too long, ventricular premature beats that occur during the AVI may not be sensed and a ventricular pacing stimulus could be delivered on to the T-wave portion of the VPB. This in turn may initiate ventricular tachyarrhythmias.

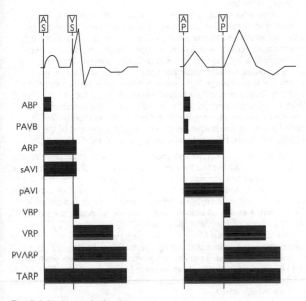

**Fig. 5.6** Blanking and refractory periods.

# Ventricular safety pacing

*Ventricular safety pacing* (VSP) is a function designed to prevent inappropriate inhibition of ventricular pacing by *far-field sensing* (crosstalk) (see 📖 p. 140) that may lead to asystole in pacing-dependent patients with dual chamber pacing modes. The ventricular safety pacing period is also known as the *ventricular triggering period* or *crosstalk sensing window*. Ventricular safety pacing is only applied following atrial paced beats as crosstalk is usually a consequence of the ventricular channel sensing the atrial pacing stimulus.

- Without ventricular safety pacing, a sensed event in the ventricular channel that occurs after the PAVB period but before the end of the pAVI will inhibit ventricular pacing as the pacemaker will assume it is an intrinsically conducted ventricular complex (Fig. 5.7(a)). This would be inappropriate if the sensed event is due to crosstalk from the atrial pacing stimulus, far-field sensing of the P wave, or artefact from ventricular lead damage. In pacing-dependent patients, inappropriate inhibition in the ventricular channel will result in asystole.
- With ventricular safety pacing, a sensed event in the ventricular channel occurring after the PAVB but before the end of the VSP period results in committed ventricular pacing at the end of the *VSP interval*, to ensure that ventricular pacing occurs (Fig. 5.7(b)).

The VSP interval is programmed shorter than the normal physiological AV delay, i.e. < 110ms, so normal, intrinsically conducted ventricular beats fall outside the interval. Any sensed events during the VSP period must therefore be due to far-field sensing of atrial stimulus or activation, ventricular premature beats, or artefact. When VSP causes a pacing spike to be delivered during an ectopic beat it will occur during the safe QRS complex and not on the vulnerable T wave.

On the surface 12-lead ECG, VSP therefore results in a shorter interval between atrial and ventricular pacing spikes (equal to the VSP interval) than one would expect from the programmed pAVI. With ventricular-based LRI timing this results in an increase in the paced rate. The AEI is calculated from the paced event delivered at the end of the VSP, not the sensed ventricular event.

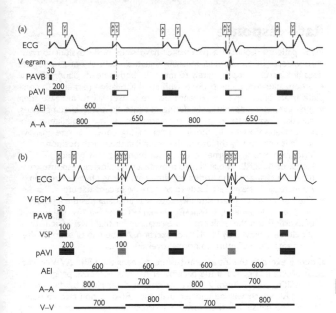

**Fig. 5.7** (a) Ventricular safety pacing off. Without ventricular safety pacing, far-field sensing of the atrial pacing spike in the ventricular channel results in a V sense, inappropriate inhibition of ventricular pacing, and begins the AEI. The next paced P wave comes earlier than expected. A ventricular premature beat occurring during atrial pacing has a similar effect, inhibiting ventricular pacing and starting the AEI and initiating the next paced P wave earlier than expected. (b) Ventricular safety pacing on. With ventricular safety pacing, if there is far-field sensing of the atrial pacing spike in the ventricular channel (after the PAVB period and during the VSP period), ventricular pacing occurs at the end of the VRP. This makes sure there is a ventricular complex. If a ventricular premature beat occurs during the VSP, the result is a further ventricular pacing spike delivered at the end of the VSP, which is before the potentially dangerous T wave.

# Rate response

Many patients requiring a pacemaker have sinus node dysfunction and chronotropic incompetence, meaning that their natural sinus node rate does not increase appropriately to meet the body's needs during physical exertion. Likewise, some patients with atrial fibrillation (either with complete heart block or a slow ventricular response) fail to increase their ventricular rates appropriately during exercise. In these circumstances, pacemakers with rate response (rate-adaptive or rate-modulating sensors) are appropriate. In the five-letter pacing code the rate-adaptive function is denoted by the use of the letter R in the fourth position.

- With rate response turned on, a sensor monitors activity and increases the LRL. The goal is to provide a physiological response to meet the change in the body's requirements during physical exertion. An increase in heart rate leads to an increase in cardiac output.
- The rate at which heart rate increases is as important as the amount of increase. In general, a response should occur within 10s of the onset of exertion and the peak heart rate required for that level of activity should be achieved by 90–120s of exertion. At the end of exercise the heart rate should return to normal over 60–120s.

If during exercise the intrinsic atrial rate exceeds the URL, AV Wenckebach occurs (📖 p. 98). If the pacemaker has rate response programmed the resulting pause during AV Wenckebach is determined by the sensor-driven LRI, which will be shorter than the LRI of a non-rate response device. The pause will therefore be shorter with rate response or may not occur if the sensor-driven URL equals the intrinsic atrial rate.

### Rate histograms

*Rate histograms* may be used to assess rate response. Heart rate ranges are divided into bins and the distribution of the number or percentage of counts is graphically presented. Paced and sensed beats are accounted for (Fig. 5.8). This allows assessment of the range of heart rates and the amount of time spent within each heart rate range. Although rate histograms indicate the range of heart rates achieved, they give little useful information regarding the sensor response.

### Trending

*Trending* is a tool that provides specific information about the sensor response. Several minutes to several hours of heart rate data can be recorded using the current rate response settings. The actual heart rate response is graphically displayed versus time and specific adjustments can then be made.

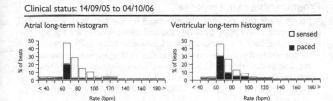

Clinical status: 14/09/05 to 04/10/06

**Fig. 5.8** Stored data recording percentage of atrial and ventricular pacing at various rates over a 13-month period.

## Rate response sensors

There are a number of sensor mechanisms used to detect increases in physical activity. The most commonly employed are *activity sensors*, *accelerometers*, and *minute ventilation sensors*.

- *Activity sensors* are piezoelectric crystals that convert movement and vibration to an electrical output. Activity that generates mechanical vibration may lead to a disproportionate increase in heart rate, whereas activity with little vibration or arm movement (cycling, swimming) may not elicit enough of a response. Also, tapping the device, or vibration from external objects such as seat-belts, may increase the paced rate even though the patient is at rest.
- *Accelerometers* use a similar principle but detect antero-posterior and vertical movement, or bending of the piezoelectric crystal within the case. These tend to offer a more predictable response and range than activity sensors, particularly at the onset of exercise.
- *Respiratory rate, tidal volume, minute ventilation* can be measured from changes in impedance between lead and pulse generator through the chest. Impedance measurements require subthreshold pacing stimulus delivered every 50ms. Transthoracic impedance increases with inspiration and decreases with expiration. Frequency of change equals the respiratory rate and amplitude the tidal volume. Minute ventilation sensing can be combined with accelerometers.
- The *intracardiac QT interval* shortens with exercise and heightened sympathetic tone. It also shortens with increased pacing rates. Measuring the QT interval from pacing spike to intracardiac T-wave peak correlates with degree of exercise and can be used to influence rate response. However, it also may be affected by undersensing or oversensing and drugs or metabolic changes.

Many modern pacemakers combine different sensors, e.g. accelerometers and minute ventilation. The two sensors may operate in a 'faster win' relationship, in which the sensor input with the fastest rate dominates, or a 'blending' relationship, in which information from both sensors is combined in a fixed ratio. Further factors, such as duration of exercise, can be used to dictate which sensor method dominates.

## Programming rate response

A pacemaker's rate response is influenced by the sensor threshold, LRI, upper sensor rate, upper tracking rate, and sensor slope. See Fig. 5.9.

- *Sensor threshold.* All sensors have a baseline 'activity' level at rest, i.e. background non-exertional vibrations, resting minute ventilation, etc. The sensor threshold is the lowest level of sensor activity that initiates an increase in heart rate above the LRI. Young, active patients usually require a higher, less sensitive threshold than older, sedentary patients.
- *Lower rate limit* (📖 p. 120). The LRL must be low enough to be appropriate for periods of rest and sleep. The sleep function can be used to facilitate this (📖 p. 96). The LRL is the baseline from which sensor activity elicits a response. The lower the LRL the greater the response required. Conventionally, an LRL of 60bpm is the nominal setting.
- *Upper sensor rate.* Physiologically, the maximum heart rate is usually calculated as (220 − age) ± 15%. Although most pacemaker recipients are elderly and require an upper rate limit no greater than 120–130bpm, younger, active patients may need values as high as 150–160 bpm. However it may not be possible to programme URLs above 150bpm without adversely affecting programmed AV delay and PVARP intervals. Also, an overly aggressive response to exertion may produce adverse symptoms of palpitations and impaired exercise capacity. The maximum sensor-driven rate (MSDR) is usually programmed equal to or faster than the maximum tracking rate. In patients exposed to a lot of vibration (e.g. Parkinson's disease) it may be appropriate to programme the sensor rate below the tracking rate.
- *Sensor slope.* The sensor slope is the rate of change of the heart rate response to increases in sensor activity. Increasing the slope will result in a faster heart rate at a particular level of activity. Unfit, inactive patients require steeper slopes than the physically fit.
- *Dynamic AV delay and dynamic PVARP.* These shorten the TARP and allow a faster URL before Wenckebach or 2:1 conduction results.

These parameters can be programmed in the pacemaker clinic by monitoring the patient's pacemaker response to simple exercise, such as walking up and down the corridor. This may be satisfactory for older, more sedentary patients. More formal chronotropic evaluation is appropriate for active patients and can be performed using an exercise treadmill with an assessment protocol. Rate modulation can be enhanced further by examining stored data in the pacemaker's diagnostic tools, if available. Rate histograms give an indication of the heart rates achieved over a set period and the level of corresponding activity.

Some devices are capable of semi-automatic and automatic programming of rate response algorithms. Optimal heart rate profiles may be determined by recording baseline profiles such as minute ventilation and then monitoring activity levels and frequency of exercise to create target rate histograms. The patient's age may also be taken into consideration by the algorithm. The device then compares actual heart rate profiles to the target profiles and adjusts the sensor parameters accordingly to obtain a good match.

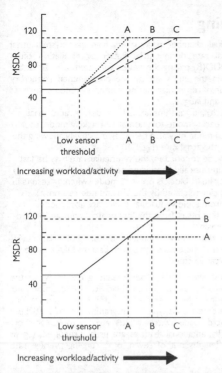

**Fig. 5.9** Rate response. Effect of alterations in the slope (top figure) and maximum sensor driven rate (MSDR, bottom figure). In the top figure, setting A has the steepest slope and the MSDR of 110bpm is reached after only a small increase in activity (suitable for younger patients). With setting C, a lot more exertion is required to reach the maximum of 110bpm (suitable for older patients). In the lower figure the slope is constant. Setting A restricts the MSDR to 95bpm after a small increase in activity and the rate cannot increase beyond this (setting suitable for patients with angina). Setting C allows for a MSDR of 140bpm, but only with extreme activity (suitable for younger, active people).

# Mode switching

Many patients with dual chamber pacemakers have paroxysmal atrial arrhythmias. The atrial rate during atrial flutter or fibrillation often exceeds 300bpm. In DDD(R) pacing the device will attempt to track the rapid atrial rate (within the limits set by the programmed refractory periods and URL). Rapid ventricular pacing causes symptoms such as palpitations, dyspnoea, and fatigue.

- Automatic *mode-switching* algorithms are used to detect rapid atrial rates and switch the pacing mode to a non-atrial tracking mode, usually VVI(R) (although DDI mode may also be used), effectively allowing the pacemaker to ignore the atrial rate (Fig. 5.10).
- If there is good AV node conduction, the ventricular rate may be fast and irregular due to intrinsically conducted beats but if AV node conduction is poor or heart block is present, mode switching results in regular ventricular pacing (dictated by the LRI and rate response).
- Symptoms resulting from rapid ventricular pacing are abolished. However symptoms that result from the loss of atrial contraction and AV synchrony will remain.
- Mode-switching algorithms allow continued monitoring of atrial activity during VVI pacing so that the device can switch back to DDD mode when the atrial tachycardia stops.

**Programming mode switching** Mode switching occurs when the sensed atrial rate exceeds a programmed atrial tachycardia detection rate. By definition, this value must be faster than the URL (maximum tracking rate). Atrial tachycardia detection is typically programmed to 175–188bpm or thereabouts. To avoid mode switching after atrial ectopics or short runs of atrial tachycardia, additional features are usually required, e.g. at least four short cycle lengths out of seven, or a running average rate (mean atrial rate).

## Mode-switching diagnostics

The frequency and duration of mode-switching episodes provide a record of atrial arrhythmia burden that can guide drug therapy and pacemaker programming. Such comprehensive monitoring in pacemaker patients has revealed that asymptomatic atrial fibrillation may occur up to 12 times more frequently than symptomatic episodes.

- *Event counters* record the number of episodes that occur. Analysis of recorded atrial EGMs indicate that 12–62% of mode-switching events are inappropriate, resulting from far-field ventricular signals. Intermittent undersensing during one long episode may trigger multiple mode switches.
- *Rate histograms* may also be useful. True AF episodes should coexist with atrial rates of > 400bpm. False episodes due to double-counting will often correspond to atrial rates of 175–250bpm. The exception to this is atrial tachycardia or flutter with an atrial rate < 250bpm.
- *Stored atrial EGMs* at the onset and offset of mode-switching episodes provide the most useful information.

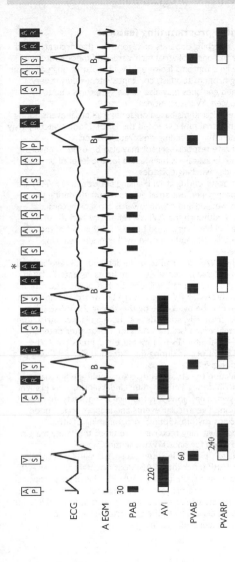

**Fig. 5.10** Mode switching. There is a paced atrial complex that conducts to the ventricle. An atrial premature beat then initiates atrial fibrillation. After 7 consecutive A–A intervals all < 333ms (180bpm) mode switching occurs (*) and the device changes to DDIR mode. Atrial sensed events falling within the PVAB are ignored (B) but those falling within the PVARP are counted (AR).

## Other mode-switch programming features

- Successful mode switching depends on algorithms that accurately and promptly identify the onset of atrial tachycardias. If mode switching happens too slowly, symptoms from rapid ventricular pacing will occur. If mode switching happens too fast, constant switches during very short non-sustained episodes may also cause symptoms due to frequent loss of paced AV association.
- Older devices used algorithms based on sensing an atrial event during the PVARP (i.e. the atrial rate exceeded the URL). Mode switching may then take less time if the preceding sinus rate is faster.
- The physiological rate response sensor may also be used to ensure that an appropriate heart rate is maintained for the level of physical activity during mode-switching episodes.
- Atrial events that occur during atrial blanking periods (e.g. PVAB) are not seen by the pacemaker, but atrial events occurring during the PVARP are acknowledged and count towards atrial tachycardia detection. Similarly, although the AVI is a refractory period, atrial events after the atrial blanking period but before the end of the AVI may be acknowledged and counted by the mode-switching algorithm in some devices.
- Blanking during the PVAB can lead to underdetection of regular atrial tachycardias such as atrial flutter. If alternate beats repeatedly fall in the PVAB the detected atrial rate will only be half of the true rate. This occurs when the AVI + PVAB is > atrial tachycardia cycle length. This phenomenon may be overcome by shortening the PVAB if it is programmable. Alternatively, some devices have a blanked atrial flutter search algorithm that extends the PVARP for 1 beat after detecting eight consecutive atrial intervals that measure < 2 times the AVI + PVAB. If an atrial event occurs during the extended PVARP the device is mode-switched (Fig. 5.11).
- During atrial fibrillation the atrial electrogram amplitude fluctuates and is often less than during sinus rhythm. Undersensing may prevent successful mode switching. However, too high a sensitivity may result in far-field detection of ventricular events and inappropriate mode switching during sinus rhythm. Optimal programming of atrial sensitivity for mode switching requires three times the safety margin compared to two times for sinus P-wave sensing.
- *Retriggerable refractory periods.* In some pacemakers an atrial signal detected in the PVARP (after the PVAB) does not start another AVI, but does initiate another TARP (AVI + PVARP). This process repeats itself. Thus, an atrial tachycardia (or sinus tachycardia) faster than the programmed upper rate effectively converts the atrial channel into an asynchronous mode, DVI(R), with the ventricular rate at the programmed LRL or sensor-driven interval.

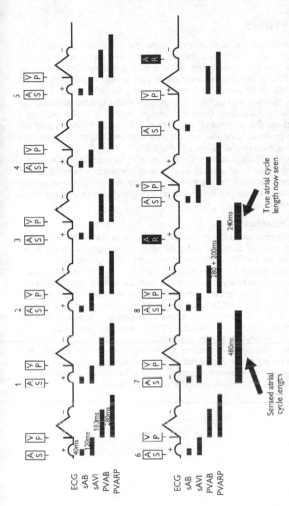

**Fig. 5.11** Flutter search algorithm. During this atrial tachycardia/flutter alternate P waves are either sensed (+) or fall within the PVAB and are not detected (–). The sensed atrial cycle length is 480ms which is < 2 times AVI + PVAB (300 x 2 = 600ms). The flutter search algorithm therefore extends the PVARP by 200ms after 8 consecutive sensed beats. This allows a P wave to fall within the PVARP and be detected, revealing the true atrial cycle length to be 240ms. Mode switching then occurs (*).

# Hysteresis

*Hysteresis* allows the rate to drop below the programmed pacing LRL, just in case an intrinsic beat arrives. If one does, pacing is inhibited. If there is no sensed event by the end of the hysteresis rate interval, pacing occurs at the faster LRL. For example, if a pacemaker is programmed VVI with an LRL of 70bpm (857ms intervals) and a hysteresis rate of 50bpm (1200ms), the pacemaker will allow the ventricular rate to fall to 50bpm before pacing. As soon as there is an escape interval of 1200ms without a sensed event the pacemaker will pace the ventricle at 70bpm and will continue to do so until the intrinsic rate exceeds 70bpm (i.e. there is a sensed event within the 857ms LRL; Fig. 5.12).

Hysteresis prolongs battery life by preventing unnecessary pacing when patients' intrinsic heart rates drop slightly below the programmed LRI. In VVI mode, hysteresis may also help maintain AV synchrony whenever possible and reduce the likelihood of retrograde conduction and pacemaker syndrome.

## Search hysteresis

*Search hysteresis* takes things a step further. Once pacing occurs, after a specific number of consecutive paced beats, the prolonged escape interval defined by the hysteresis rate is permitted. If a sensed event occurs within the prolonged escape interval, pacing is inhibited and the slow, hysteresis rate resumes. If there is no sensed event, pacing continues at the faster LRL for a further period of time. In the above example, after 256 consecutively paced beats at 70bpm, the escape interval is prolonged to 1200ms. If a sensed event occurs then pacing is inhibited and the 50bpm hysteresis rate dominates. If there is no sensed event, pacing resumes at 70bpm for another 256 beats.

In single chamber VVI systems a premature ventricular ectopic may reset the pacing rate inappropriately. In some dual chamber systems, the algorithm will only permit resetting of the hysteresis escape interval when a sensed P wave precedes the ventricular event.

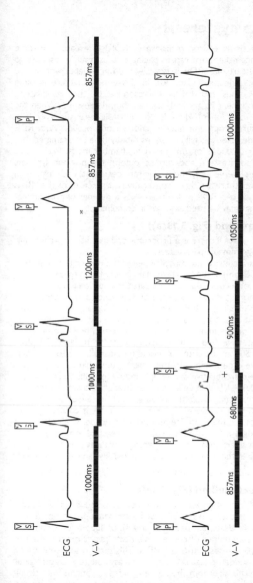

**Fig. 5.12** Hysteresis. VVI pacing with a hysteresis rate of 50bpm and LRL of 70bpm. When the V–V interval reaches 1200ms (50bpm) ventricular pacing at an LRL of 70bpm (857ms) occurs ('*'). Pacing is not inhibited until there is a sensed event within the 857ms window ('+'). When this occurs the hysteresis rate of 50bpm (1200ms) resumes.

# Rate drop hysteresis

*Rate drop hysteresis* (rate drop response or RDR) is a feature of some dual chamber pacemakers that causes pacing at a fast rate in response to a sudden fall in heart rate. RDR is typically used in patients with severe neurocardiogenic syncope (📖 p. 40). In this condition there is often an initial reflex sinus tachycardia in response to the vasodilatory, hypotensive component to try and maintain blood pressure. When the cardio-inhibitory component kicks in the intrinsic rate suddenly falls, the blood pressure drops dramatically, and syncope occurs. With RDR the pacemaker identifies this fall and paces rapidly (at a programmed rate and duration (e.g. 120bpm for 2min) in dual chamber mode. Pacing tries to maintain blood pressure and cardiac output and prevent syncope. At the end of the intervention, the pacing rate decreases, each minute, in 5–8bpm steps until there are three consecutive atrial senses or the LRL is reached. Triggering of a RDR is determined by a number of programmable algorithms that may be used alone or in combination

## Drop detect method (Fig. 5.13(a))

This algorithm is useful if there is a prodrome and initial sinus tachycardia. It uses three programmable parameters.

* *Drop rate*. Intrinsic heart rate must fall below the drop rate to initiate an RDR (e.g. 50bpm). If the heart rate falls below this rate for a programmed consecutive number of beats the criterion is satisfied. A number of consecutive beats (e.g. 2 or 3) is used to avoid post-ectopic pauses initiating a RDR. The drop rate is usually faster than the bradycardia LRL (e.g. drop rate of 50bpm with an LRL of 40 bpm).
* *Drop size*. The minimum difference in heart rate that needs to be reached in bpm (e.g. 40bpm). If the heart rate fell from 110 to 70bpm, or from 90 to 50bpm the criterion would be satisfied. The top number in the drop size is determined by the fastest rate within a programmable retrospective detection window (e.g. 30s to 2min).
* *Detection window* is used to define the top heart rate from which the drop size is calculated. When there is a gradual slowing of heart rate, a very short detection window may mean the top rate is constantly reset to slower rates and the drop size may not be reached. A very long detection window may mean the drop size is reached too easily, especially after exertion or other physiological causes of sinus tachycardia when the heart slows relatively quickly (and appropriately).

Both drop rate and drop size need to be satisfied to trigger a RDR.

## Low rate detect method (Fig. 5.13(b))

This is a simpler algorithm with a more abrupt response. The RDR is triggered if there is pacing at the LRL for more than a programmed consecutive number of beats, e.g. pacing at an LRL of 40bpm for 3 consecutive beats. Again, a number of consecutive beats (e.g. 2 or 3) is used to avoid post-ectopic pauses initiating a RDR. This rapid response is useful in patients with sudden onset bradycardia or asystole, e.g. carotid sinus hypersensitivity. This algorithm should be avoided in patients with significant resting sinus bradycardia or who require lower rate pacing.

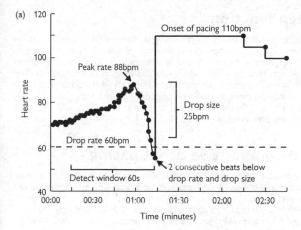

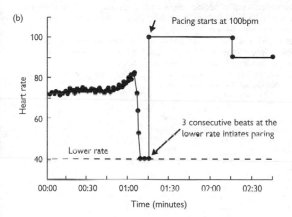

**Fig. 5.13** (a) Drop detect. Pacing at 100bpm is initiated after the drop rate criterion (heart rate < 60bpm) and drop size criterion (fall in heart rate of > 25bpm in the last 60s) are met. (b) Lower rate detect. The lower rate limit is set at 40bpm. Three consecutive paced beats at 40bpm triggers the response, which is to increase the pacing rate to 100bpm.

## Sleep function

The sleep function allows programming of different LRLs depending upon the time of day, e.g. 70bpm during waking hours and 50bpm during sleep. This may preserve battery life and also prevent the situation where sensitive patients who have heartbeat awareness when at rest notice that their heart rate is inappropriately fast when trying to get to sleep. The timer uses an internal clock. It should be remembered that, if the patient travels abroad into a different time zone, the pacemaker clock will represent their home time not their local time.

## Non-competitive atrial pacing

The *non-competitive atrial pacing* (NCAP) algorithm is used to minimize competition between the underlying sinus rate and the sensor-driven atrial paced rate.

- With NCAP disabled, If an intrinsic P wave is detected during the PVARP it is acknowledged as being in a refractory period and does not initiate an AVI. Subsequent atrial pacing may then occur at the end of the repolarization period following the ectopic (Fig. 5.14(a)). Such closely coupled atrial paced beats may initiate atrial arrhythmias such as atrial fibrillation.
- With NCAP enabled, if atrial pacing was due to occur after a preset interval (determined by the AEI or LRL) it is now delayed until a programmed time period after the detected P wave, e.g. 300ms (Fig. 5.14(b)). To maintain a more stable ventricular rate the pAVI is often shortened for that one beat.

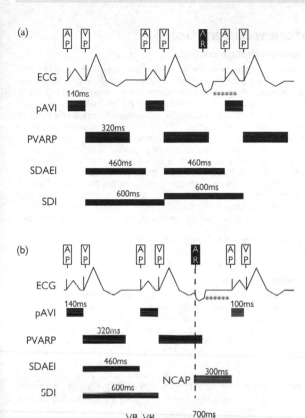

**Fig. 5.14** (a) NCAP off. The atrial premature beat falls within the PVARP and is ignored. Consequently, the next atrial paced complex is initiated shortly after the ectopic in the tail end of the atrial myocardium's refractory period (asterixes). (b) NCAP on. With NCAP, the atrial premature beat that falls within the PVARP initiates the NCAP period of 300ms, delaying the next paced atrial complex until after the atrial myocardium's refractory period is over. To lessen the impact on the ventricular rate, the pAVI is shortened. In both parts of figure: SDAEI, sensor driven atrial escape interval; SDI, sensor driven interval.

# Automated functions

## Automated capture control

The capture threshold of a pacing electrode changes with time. The ideal safety margin is a pacing output that is twice the capture threshold. Regular assessment of capture threshold may help conserve battery life by reducing pacing output or increase safety by raising it when appropriate.

Capture threshold automatically is determined by measuring the local evoked response to a stimulus. Different algorithms measure different responses (reduction in after-potential artefact or changes in the magnitude of the slew rate of the post-pacing residual lead voltage). Loss of capture is followed by an immediate high output stimulus to avoid symptomatic pauses. After determining the threshold, devices can adjust their output to a predetermined amount (e.g. twice the threshold). Modern, sophisticated devices can monitor for capture on a beat-by-beat basis that, with the addition of the loss of capture recovery, allows the output to be set to just greater than the threshold, leading to even better battery longevity.

Automated capture threshold assessment can be performed on an hourly, daily, weekly, or monthly basis. At present, only ventricular pacing leads can be reliably assessed.

## Automated sensing

As with pacing thresholds, sensing thresholds for atrial and ventricular activity change over time. Safety values are commonly set anywhere between 1/3rd and 1/6th of the sensed intrinsic electrogram amplitude (depending on whether it is atrial or ventricular). If there are a large number of consecutive relatively low or high amplitude signals the sensitivity can be increased or decreased accordingly. Other more sophisticated algorithms look at the mean of a large number of consecutive signals and compare that to the most recent EGM. They then measure the signal at the end of the ventricular refractory period, i.e. when there is no local depolarization, as a means of assessing the amplitude of background 'noise' levels.

## Other pacemaker system functional parameters

The automatic measurement of all main pacemaker system-related parameters, such as battery voltage, battery current drain, lead impedance, intrinsic signal amplitudes, ventricular pacing thresholds, and additional diagnostic data, is technically feasible. Unlike ICDs, pacemakers do not use audible alert tones when particular measurements fall outside defined parameters.

## Stored Information

## Stored information

Modern devices are able to store detailed information about patient and device activity and function. As well as information on automated testing (capture, sensing, impedance, etc.) some or all of the following information may be available (Fig. 5.15).

- Percentage of atrial and ventricular sensing and/or pacing.
- Rate histograms of atrial and ventricular paced and sensed beats.
- Average ventricular rate.
- Atrial arrhythmias (AF burden, timing, duration, and frequency of episodes).
- Ventricular high rate episodes.
- Number and timing of mode-switching episodes.
- Patient activity.
- Heart rate variability.

Depending upon the device and memory available, intracardiac EGMs can be stored during detected tachyarrhythmia events (e.g. ventricular high rate episodes, atrial tachycardia episodes) to help provide diagnostic data and rule out inappropriate detection due to far-field sensing, external noise, or lead failure.

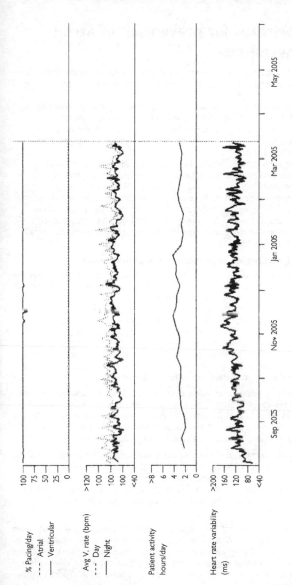

**Fig. 5.15** Stored information. Stored data recording percentage pacing, ventricular rate, activity, and heart rate variability over a 7.5 month period (Medtronic).

# Algorithms for prevention of atrial arrhythmias

Atrial arrhythmias are common in pacemaker patients, particularly those with sinus node dysfunction. There are several options to treat atrial arrhythmias.

- Treatment of sinus bradycardia with atrial pacing may in itself reduce the frequency of atrial fibrillation in a minority of individuals.
- Bradycardia pacing may allow the use of anti-arrhythmic drugs that were previously contraindicated, and this 'hybrid' therapy may be effective in some patients.
- Some sophisticated devices have additional algorithms that may be activated to prevent atrial fibrillation from occurring. It has been recognized that many paroxysmal atrial fibrillation episodes are initiated by single or multiple atrial premature beats or runs of atrial tachycardia. Sometimes this is in the setting of sinus bradycardia or post-ectopic pauses. Although prevention algorithms may reduce atrial fibrillation burden, a significant clinical impact is only found in a small number of individuals.

## Pacing strategies to prevent atrial arrhythmias

*Continuous overdrive of sinus rate at a dynamic rate (atrial overdrive pacing, atrial preference pacing)* This ensures constant atrial pacing (> 95% of the time) just above the intrinsic sinus rate. When an intrinsic sinus beat is detected the pacemaker increases the atrial LRL to 15bpm above the physiological rate. There is a gradual decrease in the LRL until a further sinus beat is detected. Premature atrial beats are ignored providing they have a short coupling interval. 'Rate smoothing' is a less aggressive variation without the large increase in heart rate. On detection of a sinus beat, the pacing rate is increased by 3bpm and decreased slowly until a further sinus beat or the lower rate limit is reached.

*Prevention of pauses that follow atrial premature beats (post-PAC response, atrial rate stabilization)* The pacemaker detects a premature atrial beat and delivers two paced beats immediately after—the first at a rate that is the average of the premature beat and the physiological sinus rate interval, the second at a rate that is the physiological sinus rate.

*Overdrive pacing at an increased atrial rate after atrial premature beats (PAC suppression)* When an atrial premature beat is sensed, the pacing rate is increased to 15bpm above the physiological rate for 600 beats. Any PACs occurring in the stable period will not induce additional rate increases. After the stable period, the atrial rate slows by 1bpm every 16 beats.

*Post-exercise response* This algorithm aims to prevent the rapid heart rate drop that can occur after exercise by enabling a temporary post-exercise rate. During exercise, the post-exercise pacing rate slowly rises to 90% of the physiological exercise rate. When the heart rate suddenly decreases after exercise, the pacemaker paces at the post-exercise pacing rate.

*Post AF response* This algorithm aims to prevent the immediate re-initiation of AF after the cessation of an earlier episode by using high rate pacing (70–100bpm for 600 beats) immediately after the arrhythmia ends.

## Pacing strategies to terminate atrial arrhythmias

It is not possible to terminate atrial fibrillation with rapid atrial overdrive pacing. Many episodes of atrial fibrillation however are preceded by a run of regular atrial tachycardia or flutter. If the atrial tachycardia can be pace-terminated the episode may be aborted before atrial fibrillation occurs.

*Atrial ramp* or *burst pacing* (at 94% of the preceding atrial cycle length) may terminate up to 54% of regular atrial tachycardias. A dual chamber device is required as appropriate ventricular detection is needed for arrhythmia discrimination purposes. Although episodes may be terminated earlier, the total atrial fibrillation burden and number of episodes may not be affected.

## Other strategies

*Alternate site atrial pacing* Dual site atrial pacing (two atrial leads, one in the right atrial appendage, the other in the low septum or coronary sinus) or single lead atrial septum/Bachmann's bundle pacing may reduce atrial fibrillation burden by providing a more homogeneous and uniform depolarization of the atria.

### Ventricular rate stabilization

As the irregular ventricular rate during atrial fibrillation impairs haemo-dynamics and contributes to symptoms and reduced cardiac output, ventricular rate stabilization algorithms have been developed to try and regularize the rhythm. The device calculates the average ventricular rate and paces the ventricle slightly faster. Concealed retrograde conduction into the AV node helps prevent antegrade activation, and blocks some atrial impulses that would otherwise have got through. The down side is that the overall rate is slightly faster and the ventricles are now activated from the RV pacing site rather than through the bundle branches, causing dyssynchrony.

# Pacemaker-mediated tachycardia

*Pacemaker-mediated tachycardia* (PMT) is also known as *endless-loop tachycardia*. It occurs with dual chamber pacemakers when a ventricular paced beat conducts retrogradely through the AV node to generate a retrograde P wave. This is sensed in the atrial channel and initiates an AVI followed by a paced ventricular beat. The paced ventricular beat again conducts retrogradely and the cycle continues indefinitely. The tachycardia often occurs at the upper rate. If the URI is longer than the TARP (AVI + PVARP) the AVI is extended by the pacemaker to conform to the URI. Pacemaker-mediated tachycardia can only occur if the retrograde P wave is sensed after the end of the PVARP. There are a number of possible events that may initiate pacemaker-mediated tachycardia.

- A ventricular premature beat that has retrograde conduction to the atrium (Fig. 5.16).
- Loss of atrial capture. There is no P wave after the atrial stimulus so the AV node and atria can be depolarized by retrograde conduction following the paced ventricular beat.
- Atrial oversensing inhibits atrial pacing so the AV node and atria can be depolarized by retrograde conduction following the paced ventricular beat.
- An atrial premature beat results in a long AV delay giving more time for the AV node and atria to recover and allow retrograde conduction after a paced ventricular beat.

Pacemaker-mediated tachycardia may also result from far-field sensing of the terminal portion of the QRS complex by the atrial channel. Thus, every paced QRS initiates an AVI followed by another paced QRS.

## Detection of pacemaker-mediated tachycardia

Automatic detection can be confirmed by the following.

- A number of consecutive paced cycles at the URL.
- A number of consecutive paced ventricular events above a programmed rate limit.
- Stability of the VP to AS interval. A constant VA time suggests retrograde VA conduction. If the pacemaker temporarily extends the sAVI for 1 beat and the VP–AS interval stays the same this suggests pacemaker-mediated tachycardia, whereas if it shortens this suggests sinus tachycardia.
- All intervals should begin with a VP event and end with an AS event.
- Use of the sensor rate can aid diagnosis, i.e. if the sensed rate is much faster than the sensor-indicated rate suggests it should be.

## Termination of pacemaker-mediated tachycardia

- Dissociation of atrial and ventricular events by inhibiting one of the ventricular stimuli.
- Dissociation of atrial and ventricular events by extension of one PVARP to include the following P wave.
- After attempts at termination there should be spontaneous atrial activity at the normal rate, atrial pacing at an appropriate rate, or redetection if there is still a tachycardia.

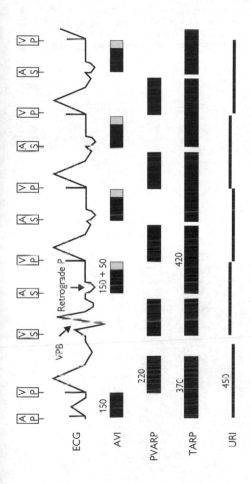

**Fig. 5.16** Pacemaker-mediated tachycardia. Pacemaker-mediated tachycardia initiated by a ventricular ectopic that conducts retrogradely through the AV node. The retrograde P wave is sensed by the atrial channel as it occurs after the PVARP, and initiates a sAVI. Ventricular pacing is subsequently conducted retrogradely and the endless loop continues. The sAVI is extended to maintain the URI and the tachycardia cycle length is at the upper rate limit.

## Avoiding pacemaker-mediated tachycardia

Pacemaker-mediated tachycardia can be avoided by programming a longer PVARP after VPBs so that the atrial channel is blanked during any retrograde atrial activation.

Unfortunately, if the next intrinsic P wave happens to fall in the PVARP it will be ignored. If it conducts to the ventricle, the intrinsic QRS is then treated as another VPB (as there is no preceding P wave) and the PVARP remains extended. This can become a repetitive cycle.

# Troubleshooting pacemakers

# General principles

Pacemakers usually fail to work appropriately due to an inability to pace or an inability to sense correctly. This may be a consequence of mechanical failure (e.g. lead fracture), surgical complications (e.g. lead displacement), or programming (incorrect pacing mode, sensitivity, or output, etc.). Other complications include diaphragmatic stimulation, muscle stimulation, tracking of atrial arrhythmias (📖 p. 112), pacemaker-mediated tachycardia (📖 p. 128), and runaway pacemaker (📖 p. 148).

## Pacing spike and the myocardial refractory period

Remember, a pacing spike delivered during the local tissue's refractory period will not result in a paced complex. This is not a failure to capture; rather it may be a failure of sensing (undersensing), appropriate pacing with fusion (📖 p. 28), inappropriate programming, or a non-sensing mode (e.g. VOO).

## The magnet

Use of a magnet may help to differentiate pacing problems from sensing problems.
- In VOO, DOO, or AOO mode, high threshold problems will remain and there will be failure to capture when the stimulus is delivered outside of the myocardial refractory period.
- If there is a sensing problem but the threshold is fine, there will be normal capture following pacing stimuli, providing they are delivered outside of the local myocardium's refractory period.

**Common reasons for failure to pace successfully**

- High threshold (pacing stimulus seen but no capture).
  - Lead displacement.
  - Lead fracture or insulation break.
  - Exit block.
  - Abnormal electrolytes/drug toxicity.
  - Scar tissue at pacing site.
- Oversensing causing inappropriate inhibition (no pacing stimulus).
  - T-wave oversensing.
  - Far-field sensing (usually R wave).
  - Myopotential inhibition.
  - Lead fracture with noise artefact.
  - Interaction with old, inactive pacing leads.
  - Lead displacement into an adjacent chamber.
- Generator failure.
  - Battery end-of-life (no pacing stimulus).

# High threshold

## Lead displacement

### Diagnosis

This typically happens in the early postoperative period. Key to diagnosis is the position of the lead on the chest radiograph (PA and lateral views, Fig. 6.1). There may be *minor* displacement, with the lead remaining in the same chamber, or *significant* displacement with the lead falling into an adjacent chamber (e.g. the atrial lead prolapsing into the right ventricle). Lead displacement may also result in a failure to sense, or inappropriate inhibition due to sensing of events in other chambers, or a pacing stimulus capturing the wrong cardiac chamber.

### Causes

Lead displacement may be a consequence of poor lead placement with insufficient 'slack' left in a lead. The lead then moves following deep inspiration or a change in posture. Alternatively, displacement may relate to the patient. 'Twiddler's syndrome' describes those patients who consciously or subconsciously fiddle with their pacemaker generator in the pocket, twisting it around. This may gradually 'wind up' the leads until they are pulled out of position (☐ p. 91). Other reasons include excessive physical activity in the early period post-implant, particularly with the arm adjacent to the generator site.

**Treatment** Lead revision is required possibly with use of active fixation leads.

---

### Atrial leads and cardiac surgery

Atrial lead displacement happens more frequently with passive fixation leads in surgically altered right atria, such as post-cardiac bypass surgery, particularly if the atrial appendage has been removed.

---

## Lead fracture

**Diagnosis** With lead fractures the stimulus may be seen on the surface ECG but fails to reach the tip of the lead and surrounding myocardium. There is usually associated failure of sensing. Key to diagnosis is an increase in the pacing impedance. A break in the lead can sometimes be seen on chest radiograph.

### Causes

The usual cause is unusual movement of the lead in a confined area. A common site for lead fracture is between the clavicle and 1st rib for leads (implanted using a standard subclavian vein puncture). The tough fascia at this site acts as a fulcrum or hinge point and repeated rubbing at this site, particularly in thicker leads, can result in 'subclavian crush syndrome'. It may be avoided by using an axillary vein (extrathoracic) puncture or cephalic cut down approach for lead insertion (☐ p. 56).

**Treatment** A new lead needs to be positioned.

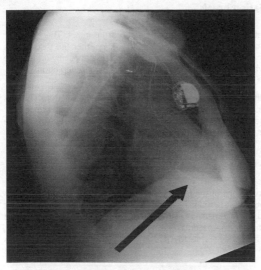

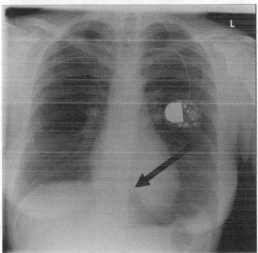

**Fig. 6.1** Atrial lead displacement. Chest radiographs (lateral and PA) showing a dual chamber pacing system with displacement of the atrial lead into the right ventricle. The black arrows show the tip of the atrial lead lying adjacent to the ventricular lead.

## Lead insulation break

### Diagnosis

Stimuli will still be present if the inner lead remains intact. There may or may not be capture of the stimuli depending on whether the threshold is increased or not. The key to diagnosis is a *decrease* in pacing impedance and excessive current loss leading to premature battery depletion.

### Causes

This is usually due to trauma to the surrounding lead insulation. This can occur at time of implant due to inadvertent damage from scalpels or scissors. Another common scenario is after elective generator change when pocket dissection causes trauma to the lead insulation.

*Treatment* A new lead is required.

## Exit block

### Diagnosis

This is due to failure of the pacing stimulus to progress beyond the electrode tip into the surrounding tissue. Diagnosis depends on excluding obvious lead displacement or lead damage and demonstrating that there is no response at the pacemaker's maximum output capacity (Fig. 6.2). There may have been a steady rise in pacing threshold over previous months.

### Causes

- Excessive fibrosis around the lead tip.
- Drugs that raise the pacing threshold (e.g. flecainide).
- Electrolyte abnormalities (hyperkalaemia, acidosis).
- Myocardial infarction involving heart tissue around the pacemaker lead tip.

### Treatment

Steroid-eluting leads have reduced the incidence of exit block by reducing fibrosis around the tip, yet it may still occur at any time even very late following lead implant. Lead revision is usually required to correct the problem.

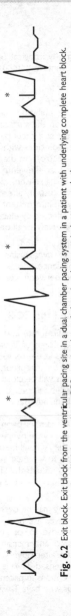

**Fig. 6.2** Exit block. Exit block from the ventricular pacing site in a dual chamber pacing system in a patient with underlying complete heart block. The ventricular pacing spikes (*) fail to result in a QRS complex. Instead, there is a slow ventricular escape rhythm.

# Oversensing

Oversensing occurs when physiological or non-physiological signals are inappropriately sensed as events and the pacemaker is inhibited.

## T-wave oversensing

### Diagnosis

This describes inappropriate inhibition due to the sensing of myocardial repolarization (represented on the surface ECG by the T wave). Confirmation of the diagnosis requires a pacemaker programmer (Fig. 6.3).

- Ventricular sense marker coincides with T wave on surface ECG.
- On the ventricular lead electrogram the local T-wave repolarization amplitude will be greater than the ventricular channel sensitivity setting (hence the reason for it being sensed).
- Sensed ventricular intervals usually alternate, with R–T < T–R interval.
- T-wave oversensing may be intermittent as T-wave morphology and size can be dynamic and affected by electrolytes and drugs.
- It may occur following relatively small or large R waves (Fig. 6.4).

**Causes** Surface ECG amplitude and local T-wave measurements are dynamic. Therefore T-wave oversensing can start to occur following ischaemia, electrolyte imbalance, drugs, and exercise. Local T-wave amplitude may also differ between ventricular paced and ventricular sensed events.

### T-wave oversensing and the ECG

Although diagnosis is confirmed using the pacemaker programmer, there are characteristic ECG signs of T-wave oversensing.
- In VVI mode the LRI starts at the sensed ventricular event. Therefore, the distance from inappropriately sensed T wave to next ventricular pacing stimulus will be close to the LRI. This means the ventricular paced rate will be slower than the programmed LRL because the interval will include the time from ventricular event to T wave.
- In ventricular-based dual chamber pacing the AEI is initiated by a sensed ventricular event. T-wave oversensing therefore results in a delay in atrial pacing as the AEI will be timed from the T wave. The distance from the T wave to the next atrial pacing stimulus will be close to the AEI (which equals the LRI – AVI). The overall ventricular rate will be slower than the programmed LRL.

**Treatment** T-wave oversensing may be overcome by decreasing ventricular channel sensitivity until T waves are no longer sensed. A problem arises when T-wave amplitude is close to, or greater than, R-wave amplitude. Decreased sensitivity leads to undersensing of ventricular depolarization and inappropriate pacing. An alternative strategy is to lengthen the VRP until it extends beyond the sensed T-wave component in the local EGM. Although both are sensible options in pacemakers, they must be used with caution in patients with ICDs who have T-wave oversensing (📖 p. 258).

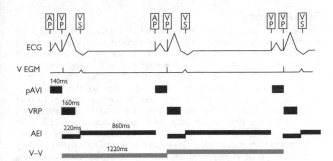

**Fig. 6.3** T-wave oversensing. T-wave oversensing in a dual chamber pacemaker. Following ventricular pacing the ventricular electrogram (V EGM) shows the repolarization component is large enough to be sensed by the pacemaker (VS). It falls after the VRP so is not blanked. This resets the AEI, delaying the next atrial stimulus by 220ms, reducing the overall paced rate to 49bpm (1220ms), which is below the programmed LRL of 60bpm (1000ms).

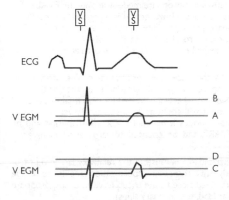

**Fig. 6.4** Reprogramming options for T-wave oversensing. In the top example the R wave is considerably bigger than the sensed T-wave, so changing the sensitivity from A to B avoids T-wave oversensing while maintaining a good safety margin. In the lower example the R wave is only just greater than the T-wave. Changing the sensitivity from C to D risks undersensing ventricular R waves. It would be more appropriate to extend the VRP to blank the sensed T wave.

### Far-field sensing

This describes local sensing, in the atrium or ventricle, of events from the other cardiac chamber. This is more common with unipolar pacing systems. Far-field sensing of atrial activity in the ventricular channel is rare and usually means the lead has displaced or has been incorrectly positioned in the coronary sinus. Typically, the atrial channel *far-field senses* ventricular depolarization (R waves) due to the significantly greater myocardial mass of the ventricles. In some cases, the far-field R wave amplitude may be greater than the local atrial electrogram, particularly if the atrial lead is near the tricuspid valve. Far-field R-wave sensing may inappropriately inhibit atrial pacing and is therefore of particular concern when atrial pacing is required (AAI or DDD pacing modes). It may also result in inappropriate mode-switching by double counting and falsely detecting atrial arrhythmias (Fig. 6.5).

---

#### Mode switching and far-field sensing

- If the far-field R-wave sensing falls within the PVARP and mode-switching algorithms are being used it may result in inappropriate mode switching by double-counting the true atrial rate.
- If far-field sensing causes inappropriate *mode-switching*, the PVAB period should be lengthened. However, if it is extended out too far it decreases the device's ability to detect appropriately atrial fibrillation and also means regular atrial tachycardias (e.g. atrial flutter) are more likely to be tracked at a 2:1 ventricular rate.

---

*Diagnosis* is made with the pacemaker programmer. The atrial event marker will coincide inappropriately with ventricular events (or the ventricular event marker with atrial activity). In AAI mode if it falls outside of the atrial blanking period it will count as a sensed atrial event and reset the LRI. In dual chamber modes it may fall in the PVAB period and be ignored, or in the PVARP and be counted towards atrial tachycardia detection.

*Causes* This may be unavoidable because of the relatively larger ventricular amplitude, due to dynamic changes in repolarization amplitudes or due to lead placement (atrial lead close to the tricuspid valve or inappropriate placement of ventricular lead, e.g. coronary sinus).

#### Treatment

- In *single chamber* AAI systems, far-field R-wave sensing in the atrial channel may be overcome by extending the atrial blanking or refractory periods (ABP or ARP).
- In *dual chamber* systems the PVAB or PVARP should be extended to prevent far-field R wave sensing in the atrial channel.

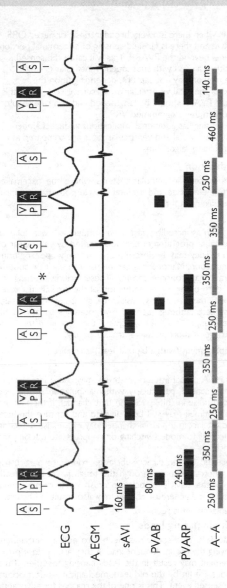

**Fig. 6.5** Far-field R waves. DDD pacing with atrial sensing and ventricular pacing. The far-field R wave is sensed in the atrial channel after the PVAB period has completed. As it falls within the PVARP no sAVI is initiated, but there is double counting in the atrial channel with alternating atrial intervals of 250ms and 350ms (rather than the true interval of 600ms). This satisfies the programmed criteria for mode-switching (*) which switched the pacemaker to VVI mode.

- A rare variation is when there is a very broad intrinsic or paced QRS complex or T wave and there is far-field sensing of its terminal portion in the atrial channel beyond the PVARP. This will cause the sensed atrial event to initiate an AVI with subsequent ventricular pacing. The pacing spike may or may not capture, depending upon the refractory period of the local ventricular myocardium. To prevent this from occurring the PVARP should be lengthened and as a rule should always be longer than the programmed VRP.
- Far-field R wave sensing has additional implications in dual chamber ICDs, particularly when atrial and ventricular rates are compared as part of SVT discriminator algorithms.

## Myopotential inhibition

This is a complication seen in unipolar systems where the pacemaker generator is an active electrode and skeletal muscle potentials inappropriately inhibit pacemaker output.

### Diagnosis

Myopotentials are seen as incredibly fast, high frequency, low amplitude signals on the pacemaker programmer that are marked by ventricular or atrial event markers. They may be intermittent and only appear during skeletal muscle contraction. Manoeuvres can be used to elicit myopotentials and demonstrate inappropriate sensing. These include pressing the hands hard against each other, hyper adduction of the arm against resistance, lifting or flexing the arm against resistance, sit-ups, or if necessary, a treadmill exercise test. Although sensed myopotentials usually inhibit pacing in the same channel, in DDD systems if they occur in the atrial channel they may trigger inappropriate ventricular pacing.

**Treatment** Lead replacement (with a bipolar lead) is required.

## Lead fracture

**Diagnosis** (📖 p. 134) A partial fracture or break may cause intermittent noise artefacts to be sensed, particularly with manipulation of the lead (Fig. 6.6). The sensed noise inhibits pacing in that channel. If the fracture is partial then pacing stimuli may still be delivered and capture the local myocardium. Noise artefact in the atrial channel may cause false detection of high atrial rates leading to mode switching or inappropriate tracking and pacing in the ventricle.

**Causes** Leads implanted by the direct subclavian route are particularly prone to fracture where they pass through the tough fascia underneath the medial aspect of the clavicle (subclavian crush syndrome). Trauma from sports, accidents, and generator change may also result in fracture.

**Treatment** Lead replacement is required.

## Interaction with old pacing leads

If a pacemaker lead fails, it is sometime elected to add a replacement lead without removing the old, redundant lead. If they are in close proximity, cardiac movement may result in the leads banging together. If the new lead's electrodes are hit by the old lead, mechanical artefact occurs that may result in a sensed event. This is one of the reasons for advocating extraction of redundant leads, particularly in ICDs (📖 p. 328).

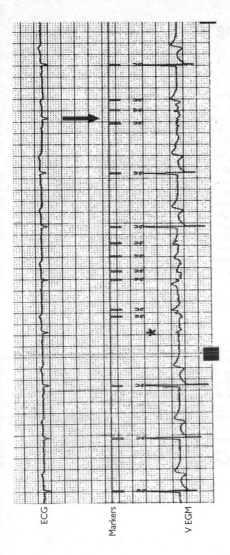

**Fig. 6.6** Lead fracture. The first 3 ventricular complexes are sensed appropriately with large R waves in the electrogram. The device is then gently manoeuvred in the pocket, revealing the presence of a lead fracture with failure to sense (* and arrow) and noise artefact that registers as ventricular sensed events (VS).

ECG

Markers

V EGM

# Undersensing

Pacemakers may act inappropriately by delivering a pacing spike when one should not occur. If delivered because there has been no inhibition when inhibition should have occurred, the fault may be *undersensing*. The pacing spike may or may not result in capture of local myocardium, depending upon whether the myocardium at the pacing lead tip is refractory (Fig. 6.7(a)). Common reasons for inappropriate pacing are:

• undersensing due to small local signals;
• undersensing due to events falling into blanking or refractory periods;
• battery end-of-life (ERI features, e.g. VOO mode).

*Undersensing* refers to the failure of a device to respond to an appropriate signal occurring during the alert (i.e. non-refractory) period of a timing cycle. Failure to detect the signal means there is no inhibition when inhibition should occur; thus a pacing spike is delivered when it is not required. This may in turn influence further timing cycles, such as the AEI, AVI, etc. In rare instances, undersensing may result in delivery of a ventricular pacing spike in the middle of the T-wave (R-on-T) which can result in dangerous ventricular arrhythmias. Undersensing of atrial tachycardias such as atrial fibrillation may occur as the atrial electrogram amplitude is usually smaller during fibrillation than during sinus rhythm. This can result in a failure to mode switch appropriately (Fig. 6.7(b)).

## Diagnosis

The ECG will show delivery of pacing spikes when they should be inhibited by intrinsic events. If there is a significant lead problem, there may also be failure to capture even when the pacing spike is delivered (assuming the myocardium has recovered and is no longer refractory). A CXR may reveal lead displacement or fracture. Pacemaker interrogation with simultaneous ECG recording will demonstrate failure to sense intrinsic events and to determine whether it is a true sensing failure or a functional problem as a consequence of pacemaker programming. The current amplitudes of intrinsic events should be measured through the programmer and manually on paper printouts. These can be compared with current sensitivity settings. The measured EGM amplitudes at implant should be reviewed, bearing in mind that the rhythm at implant (atrial fibrillation, temporary ventricular pacing) may be different from the current underlying rhythm. The programmer will also indicate whether events are falling into refractory or blanking periods.

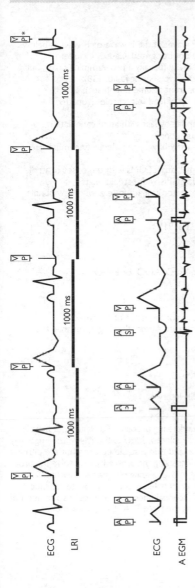

**Fig. 6.7** (a) Ventricular lead undersensing. There is a single chamber VVI pacemaker that is undersensing the ventricular R wave. Ventricular pacing is therefore not inhibited and pacing spikes are delivered at 1000ms (60bpm) intervals, despite sinus rhythm with intact AV conduction occurring at a faster rate. When a pacing spike falls on fully recovered myocardium it results in a paced QRS complex; when it falls on the T wave the myocardium is still refractory and there is no capture (*). (b) Undersensing of atrial fibrillation. There are two paced atrial complexes. There is then a sensed atrial ectopic beat (that initiates a sAVI and paced QRS) that triggers atrial fibrillation. The amplitude of the fibrillatory waves is not large enough to be detected with the atrial sensitivity setting (grey line) so there is no mode-switching and there is inappropriate atrial pacing which does not elicit a P wave.

**Causes**
- Small intrinsic R waves or P waves. If the P wave or R wave is below the sensitivity setting, it will not be sensed. Causes include:
  - inappropriately low sensitivity (usually a programming error, but may be deliberate to avoid oversensing 📖 p. 138);
  - poor contact (usually apparent at time of implant);
  - diseased myocardium at tip of lead (e.g. cardiomyopathy, myocardial infarction);
  - previous surgery (e.g. cardiac bypass with atrial cannulation);
  - tip fibrosis and lead maturation;
  - medications (class I anti-arrhythmics) and electrolyte imbalance (hyperkalaemia);
  - change in rhythm (e.g. small atrial EGMs with the onset of atrial fibrillation, low amplitude EGMs with ectopic beats);
  - change in depolarization vector at lead tip (e.g. with new bundle branch block).
- Lead dislodgment:
  - 'twiddler's syndrome' (📖 p. 91);
  - poor position at implant.
- Lead failure:
  - insulation break.
- Pacemaker mode change to VOO, AOO, or DOO:
  - ERI feature;
  - magnet application;
  - noise reversion.
- Functional undersensing (i.e. a consequence of pacemaker programming, not electrogram amplitude, that is greater than the sensitivity setting):
  - PMT intervention;
  - safety pacing;
  - PVARP extension post-PVC;
  - long PVARP and high LRL;
  - fast sinus rate and long PR interval.

**Treatment**
Treatment is directed at the underlying problem. For lead dislodgment or fracture the lead needs to be replaced. New anti-arrhythmic drugs may need to be discontinued. If the lead is in a stable position but the intrinsic electrogram amplitude is low, increasing the sensitivity may solve the problem as long as it does not result in oversensing of other activity (e.g. far-field R or T waves) which would in turn lead to inappropriate inhibition or mode-switching (📖 p. 138). Functional undersensing requires alteration of programmed parameters such as the PVARP, AVI, or pacing mode.

# Generator failure

Generators very rarely fail due to electronic or mechanical problems. A generator usually stops working because the battery has run out.

### Battery end-of-life

At the end of life (EOL) complete battery failure results in loss of pacemaker sensing and pacing. This should be evident from the pacemaker programmer although complete generator failure may make it impossible to interrogate the device. ERI features will be present in pacemaker checks before this stage. Generator replacement is required.

### Runaway pacemaker

Now very rare to see, runaway pacemaker is a generator malfunction causing the pacemaker to pace incessantly at its maximum rate. Modern devices usually have a 'runaway protection circuit' limiting the maximum pacing rate to 150–180bpm. With generator failure it may be impossible to interrogate and reprogramme the device. Generator replacement is required.

# Diaphragmatic stimulation

## Diagnosis

Diaphragmatic stimulation causes a distressing twitch or hiccup of the diaphragm may be constant or intermittent and be related to posture and respiration. The twitching coincides with a pacing stimulus. Pacing at maximum output (usually 10V and 2.0ms) should have been performed at implant to ensure this does not occur. If it first occurs during follow-up it usually indicates lead movement or slight perforation.

## Treatment

Reducing the pacing output may limit diaphragmatic stimulation. Ensure there is still an adequate safety margin; otherwise there may be failure to pace. If this is not possible, lead revision may be required.

# Skeletal muscle stimulation

A rare complication that may occur in unipolar systems, pectoral muscle stimulation may occur if there is an insulation break in a pacing lead along its proximal, extra-thoracic course. The gap in lead insulation allows direct contact and stimulation of surrounding skeletal muscle that can cause chest wall twitching. A perforating right ventricular lead that extends beyond the pericardial space may cause direct intercostal muscle stimulation.

## Treatment

Reducing the pacing output may limit muscle stimulation but if the under-lying cause is insulation break or perforation lead revision is likely to be required.

# Pacemaker-mediated tachycardia

Pacemaker-mediated tachycardia (aka. endless-loop tachycardia) is an incessant tachycardia in dual chamber tracking modes with ventricular pacing and atrial sensing usually at the pacemaker's upper rate limit. It results from retrograde conduction of paced ventricular complexes up through the AV node with a retrograde P wave that occurs after the end of the PVARP. The P wave is sensed in the atrial channel and initiates an AVI and subsequent paced ventricular complex and the cycle continues (📖 p. 128).

## Diaphragmatic stimulation and leads

- *Right atrial lead.* If placed on the lateral border of the right atrium, atrial pacing may cause stimulation of the right phrenic nerve with twitching of the right hemidiaphragm.
- *Right ventricular lead.* If the inferior wall of the right ventricle is very thin, or the tip of the right ventricular lead penetrates into the myocardium or perforates through it, there may be direct stimulation of the right hemidiaphragm.
- *Left ventricular pacing lead.* A common complication of biventricular pacing is stimulation of the left phrenic nerve where it runs over the epicardial surface of the lateral left ventricular wall. This results in twitching of the left hemidiaphragm.

# Suspected pacemaker malfunction with and without visible pacing stimuli on ECG

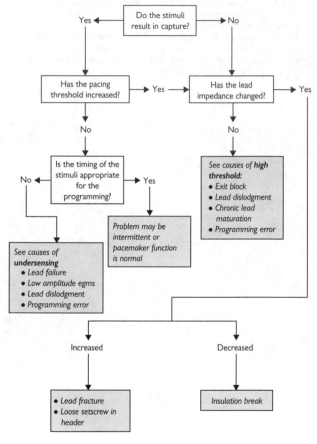

**Fig. 6.8** Suspected pacemaker malfunction with visible pacing stimuli on ECG.

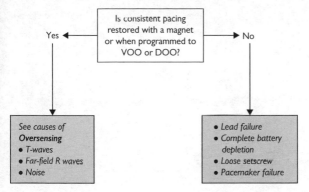

**Fig. 6.9** Suspected pacemaker malfunction without visible pacing stimuli on ECG.

# Temporary cardiac pacing

# General principles

Recommendations for temporary pacing are based on consensus of clinical opinion rather than trial data. If a patient requires a permanent pacemaker, if at all possible a temporary wire should be avoided and a permanent system implanted. Patients requiring a permanent system should only undergo temporary pacing for syncope at rest, haemodynamic compromise, or bradycardia-induced ventricular tachyarrhythmias. Sinus node disease rarely requires temporary pacing.

The indications can be split into two broad categories: emergency (commonly with acute MI) and semi-elective. In acute anterior MI, complete heart block is associated with a poor prognosis, associated with a broad QRS and represents tissue necrosis in the His–Purkinje system. Complete heart block in acute inferior MI is usually reversible, associated with a narrow QRS, and may respond to atropine.

## Risk of 3rd degree AV block after infarction

The MILIS (Multicentre Investigation of the Limitation of Infarct Size) study has recommended a method of risk stratification for the development of 3rd degree AV block following myocardial infarction.[1] One point is scored for each of the following:
• 1st degree AV block;
• type I 2nd degree AV block;
• type II 2nd degree AV block;
• left anterior fascicular block;
• left posterior fascicular block;
• right bundle branch block;
• left bundle branch block.

The risk of 3rd degree AV block is predicted by the score as follows.

| Score | Risk of 3rd degree AV block (%) |
|-------|--------------------------------|
| 0 | 1.2 |
| 1 | 7.8 |
| 2 | 25 |
| 3 | 36.4 |

## Reference

1 Lamas GA, Muller JE, Turi ZG, et al. (1986). A simplified method to predict occurrence of complete heart block during acute myocardial infarction. *Am J Cardiol* **57** (15), 1213–19.

# ACC/AHA guidelines[2]

## Emergency

### Acute MI (class I—good evidence for benefit)
- Asystole.
- Symptomatic bradycardia (sinus bradycardia with hypotension and type I second degree AV block not responsive to atropine).
- Bilateral bundle branch block (alternating BBB or RBBB with alternating LAHB/LPHB).
- New or indeterminate age bifascicular block with 1st degree AV block.
- Mobitz type II second degree AV block.

### Bradycardia not associated with acute MI
- Asystole.
- 2nd or 3rd degree AV block with haemodynamic compromise.
- Ventricular tachyarrhythmias secondary to bradycardia.

### Acute MI (class IIa/b—some evidence for benefit)
- RBBB with LAFB or LPFB (new or indeterminate).
- RBBB with 1st degree AV block.
- LBBB (new or indeterminate).
- Recurrent sinus pauses (> 3s); not responsive to atropine.
- Incessant VT for overdrive pacing.
- Bifascicular block of indeterminate age.
- RBBB.

## Semi-elective
- Support for procedures that may promote bradycardia.
- General anaesthesia with:
  - 2nd or 3rd degree AV block;
  - intermittent AV block;
  - 1st degree AV block and bifascicular block;
  - 1st degree AV block and LBBB.
- Cardiac surgery:
  - aortic surgery;
  - tricuspid surgery;
  - VSD closure;
  - ostium primum ASD repair.
- Rarely considered for PCI (usually right coronary artery).

## Reference
2 Gregoratos G, Abrams J, Epstein AE, *et al.* (2002). ACC/AHA/NASPE 2002 guideline update for implantation of cardiac pacemakers and antiarrhythmia devices: summary article: a report of the American College of Cardiology/American Heart Association Task Force on Practice Guidelines (ACC/AHA/NASPE Committee to Update the 1998 Pacemaker Guidelines). *Circulation* **106** (16), 2145–61.

# Preparation for transvenous temporary pacing

As with all techniques preparation is important before starting a procedure. Ensure the following are available or set up before starting.

## Equipment

- Peripheral IV access.
- 3 lead ECG monitoring (avoid leads on the chest that may obscure screening).
- Transcutaneous external pacing accessible, if available.
- Sterile drapes, gown, and gloves.
- Iodine skin preparation or equivalent.
- Lidocaine for local anaesthesia.
- Introducer sheath with haemostatic valve (usually 6F and at least one size larger than the electrode).
- Temporary pacing electrode (semi-rigid or flotation).
- Temporary pulse generator.
- Connecting leads for pacing box to the electrode.
- Suture material and scalpel for sheath and the electrode.
- Transparent occlusive dressing.
- X-ray equipment and operator.

## Patient preparation

- Patients need to be on a dedicated pacing bed in order to accept the C-arm of the X-ray equipment.
- Sedation is usually not required.
- The patient should be slightly head down.
- Select venous access site (subclavian, internal jugular, or femoral) and side of access (left or right).
- Reposition any transcutaneous pacing leads or ECG monitoring electrodes that are too close to the access site.
- Once you have scrubbed up, prepare the skin in the venous access area, usually with an iodine-based surgical wash. If subclavian or internal jugular access is to be used prepare both sites so that either can be used without the need to re-prepare the patient if one fails.
- Position appropriate sterile drapes around the venous access site and fix with clips, if available.
- Infiltrate the access site with local anaesthetic, e.g. lidocaine 1%.

## Choice of venous access

The choice of access is often dependent on individual experience but consideration should also be given to the length of time for which it is anticipated that the temporary wire will be needed.

- Current BCS guidelines recommend the right internal jugular vein route as this is felt to be more stable over longer periods and can be kept sterile.
- Subclavian access is a familiar approach for those who regularly perform permanent pacing but there is a higher risk of pneumothorax.
- In an emergency situation where immediate pacing is required (e.g. no transcutaneous pacing available) the femoral route is often easiest for both access and lead positioning. Bleeding can also be easily controlled with pressure and therefore is useful in the anticoagulated or thrombolysed patient. However, over the longer term femoral pacing wires restrict patient mobility, are more liable to displace, and less easy to keep clean.
- If available, ultrasound guidance can be used to gain central venous access.

# Internal jugular vein cannulation

The right internal jugular approach (Fig. 7.1) offers the most direct route to the right ventricle and has the lowest complication and highest success rate. Compared to subclavian approach it has a reduced risk of pneumothorax and allows for direct compression for haemostasis if bleeding occurs. The left internal jugular should be avoided due to the angulation required and the presence of the thoracic duct.

- Prepare and drape the skin; position patient in slight head-down position (📖 p. 160).
- Identify the apex of the triangle between the clavicular and manubrial heads of sternocleidomastoid.
- Infiltrate the skin and subcutaneous tissue with around 10mL of lidocaine 1–2%.
- Some people like to nick the skin with a small (e.g. no. 11) scalpel blade at the planned point of entry. Alternatively, this can be done once the wire has been passed into the vein.
- Palpate the line of the carotid artery and insert the needle with syringe attached lateral to this line at an angle of 45° to the skin, aiming for the right nipple area (or anterior superior iliac spine).
- Advance the needle slowly with some negative pressure on the syringe so that venous blood is withdrawn when the vein is cannulated. The vein is superficial and cannulation should be achieved at a depth of a few cm. Do not advance beyond this as the apex of the lung could be injured. Some people initially identify the position of the vein with a small gauge needle before using the needle for cannulation.
- When venous access is obtained, remove the syringe and pass the wire down through the needle. If the wire does not pass freely then do not force the wire. Withdraw the wire and ensure you can still pull back blood from the needle. It may have moved position.
- Once the wire is in place remove the needle, nick the skin (if not already done), and pass the dilators over the wire. Then introduce the haemostatic sheath and remove the wire.

### Difficult internal jugular access

- If you accidentally access the carotid artery, firm pressure will be needed for a number of minutes to obtain haemostasis. A large haematoma may make access to the internal jugular difficult.
- If you cannot get access try an alternative (femoral or subclavian) and consider getting senior help.

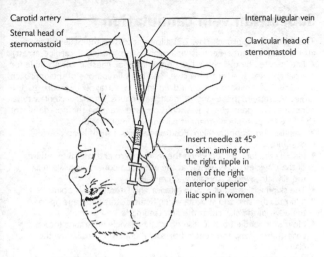

Carotid artery

Sternal head of
sternomastoid

Internal jugular vein

Clavicular head of
sternomastoid

Insert needle at 45°
to skin, aiming for
the right nipple in
men of the right
anterior superior
iliac spin in women

**Fig. 7.1** Right internal jugular vein cannulation.

# Subclavian vein cannulation

The subclavian approach (Fig. 7.2) allows access to the patient if the area around the patient's head is unavailable (e.g. during a cardiac arrest). A line inserted by this route lies on the anterior chest, is comfortable for the patient, and is easy to manage. The main limitations of the approach are a risk of pneumothorax and an inability to apply pressure to the target vessels in the event of multiple venous or inadvertent arterial puncture. The dominant side should be used, keeping the non-dominant side free for possible permanent pacemaker implantation.

- Prepare and drape the skin. Position patient in slight head-down position.
- Identify the junction between the medial third and lateral two-thirds of the clavicle (this is usually at the apex of a convex angulation as the clavicle sweeps laterally and cranially).
- The skin incision point is 2cm inferior and lateral to this point.
- Infiltrate the skin and subcutaneous tissue at this point and up to the edge of the clavicle at the first landmark.
- Move the needle tip stepwise down the clavicle infiltrating local anaesthetic. Keep the needle horizontal until it moves below the clavicle.
- Prepare the cannulation needle and follow the same initial track as the anaesthetic needle.
- When the needle lies just below the clavicle swing the needle round to aim at the nadir of the suprasternal notch.
- Keeping the needle horizontal and parallel to the bed (avoiding lifting the hands off the body and angling the needle tip down) minimizes the risk of pneumothorax.
- Advance the needle slowly with some negative pressure on the syringe so that venous blood is withdrawn when the vein is cannulated.
- When venous access is obtained, remove the syringe and pass the wire down through the needle. If the wire does not pass freely then do not force the wire. Withdraw the wire and ensure you can still pull back blood from the needle. (It may have moved position).
- Once the wire is in place remove the needle, nick the skin (if not already done), and pass the dilators over the wire. Then introduce the haemostatic sheath and remove the wire.

### Difficult subclavian access

- If you have failed to get access on one side *do not* attempt subclavian access on the other side due to the risk of bilateral iatrogenic pneumothoraces.
- If you cannot get access try an alternative (femoral or internal jugular) and consider getting senior help.

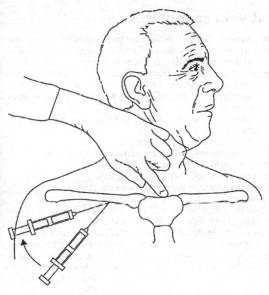

**Fig. 7.2** Right subclavian vein puncture.

# Femoral vein cannulation

The femoral approach (Fig. 7.3) allows easy cannulation of a great vein and is valuable in an emergency setting. The area can be compressed in the event of bleeding and as such is probably the access of choice in the setting of thrombolysis. The main limitations relate to subsequent patient immobility and a probable increased risk of line infection. There is also an increased risk of deep vein thrombosis with a temporary wire in place for a prolonged period.

- The patient should be lying flat with the leg slightly adducted and externally rotated.
- Shave the groin, prepare the skin, and drape.
- Palpate the femoral artery below the inguinal ligament, over or slightly above the natural skin crease at the top of the leg.
- The femoral vein lies medial to the femoral artery.
- Infiltrate local anaesthetic at the skin surface over the femoral vein and deeper layers.
- Advance the cannulation needle at 30–45° to the skin surface. The vein usually lies ~2–4cm from the skin surface.
- Advance the needle slowly with some negative pressure on the syringe so that venous blood is withdrawn when the vein is cannulated.
- When venous access is obtained, remove the syringe and pass the wire down through the needle. If the wire does not pass freely then do not force the wire. Withdraw the wire and ensure you can still pull back blood from the needle. (It may have moved position.)
- Once the wire is in place remove the needle, nick the skin (if not already done), and pass the dilators over the wire. Then introduce the haemostatic sheath and remove the wire.

## Difficult femoral access

- The femoral vein is often more medial than one thinks.
- The right femoral is easier to access for most operators.
- If the guide wire or sheath will not advance, screen at the groin to confirm wire position. It may pass into the contralateral femoral vein or even distally into the leg if the puncture is vertical.

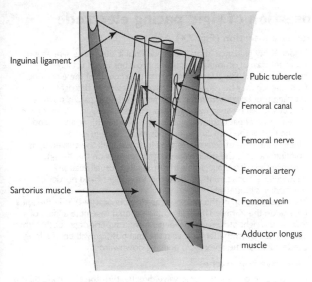

**Fig. 7.3** Right femoral vein anatomy.

# Insertion of rigid pacing electrode

## Standard insertion (Fig. 7.4)

- Under X-ray guidance insert electrode until it sits in the right atrium.
- From subclavian or internal jugular approaches this is usually straightforward. For a femoral approach, screening of the electrode from the leg may be required to ensure it passes to the right atrium avoiding tributaries within the abdomen. If the lead passes down a tributary it will be seen heading away from the midline or curving over (often into a hepatic tributary under the diaphragm). A small bend on the end of the lead can sometimes make passage easier.
- Once in the right atrium rotate the electrode until the curved tip is pointing towards the tricuspid valve (to the right on the X-ray).
- Advance the wire through the tricuspid valve (usually causing ventricular ectopics) until it sits at the apex (right-hand border of the cardiac silhouette).
- Manipulate the tip of the wire so that it points downwards in the apex (lateral on the X-ray). The final position should resemble a 'heel of a foot' in the right atrium when viewed from a superior approach. When approached from the femoral vein the final position will be of a long gentle curve to the apex again pointing downwards.

## Alternative approaches

- If unable to cross the tricuspid valve directly, turn the electrode till it is pointing towards the free wall of the right atrium (left on the X-ray). Advance the wire with the tip pressing against the free wall and try to form a loop in the right atrium. This may then spontaneously prolapse across the tricuspid valve. Alternatively, slight rotation of the electrode may flick the tip into the right ventricle
- Once in the ventricle manipulate the electrode and aim for the tip to lie in the apex as described above.

### Difficult electrode positioning

- Inadvertent positioning in the coronary sinus results in a lead pointing up and to the patient's left. Compared to a position in the RVOT on pulling the lead back and rotating it will only follow back in the same line (with a lead in the RVOT it will flop downwards into the cavity of the RV).
- Sensing in the coronary sinus shows a large P wave and QRS.
- The tip of most rigid electrodes can be moulded to change the angle of the tip if crossing the tricuspid valve is problematic.
- If all attempts with a rigid electrode fail change to a flotation electrode.
- With severe tricuspid regurgitation the electrode may repeatedly 'blow' back into the right atrium. This can be a difficult situation. It may require positioning of a permanent active lead and occasionally the use of a CS sheath (normally used for CRT pacing).

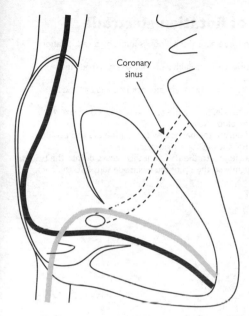

Coronary
sinus

**Fig. 7.4** Position of temporary pacing wire. View of pacing wire in the right ventricular apex from an upper approach (black) and femoral approach (grey). Note the coronary sinus running in the posterior portion of the atrioventricular groove.

# Insertion of flotation electrode

- Before insertion make sure the balloon is intact by a test inflation (Fig. 7.5).
- Under X-ray guidance, if available, advance the electrode into the right atrium.
- Inflate the balloon with 1mL of air and lock into the balloon by turning the tap.
- Advance the electrode. Ideally the balloon is dragged across the tricuspid valve by blood flow.
- Once in the RV deflate the balloon by turning the tap and position the lead in the RV apex as for a rigid electrode.
- The balloon may float into the RVOT. If this occurs deflate the balloon and pull back slightly so the tip of the electrode slips into the apex.

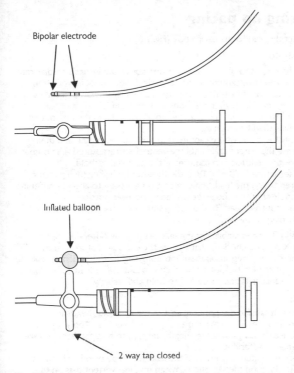

**Fig. 7.5** Flotation temporary pacing electrode with balloon deflated and inflated.

# Setting up pacing

Connect the lead to the pacing box (Fig. 7.6).

## Threshold

- Set the output to 3V and pace at a rate above the intrinsic cardiac rate.
- Ensure you have capture of the ventricle. If not, check all your lead connections and that the pacing box is properly powered. If still no capture, reposition your electrode and try again.
- If there is capture of the ventricle, slowly turn down the box output watching the ECG monitor.
- Identify the point where capture is lost. Note the output and then increase the output again until the ventricle is recaptured. The output where the ventricle is recaptured is the pacing threshold.
- Aim for a threshold of < 1V. If the threshold is higher then go back and reposition the lead. Sometimes it is necessary to accept borderline thresholds but this should be avoided wherever possible.
- Set output to at least 3× the pacing threshold to ensure a good safety margin.

**Stability** Test the stability of the lead position by observing lead motion on the X-ray and checking that the ventricle is still captured on the ECG monitor during deep inspiration and coughing (if the patient is able to comply). If the lead is not stable then reposition the lead (often just by gently advancing it) and recheck threshold and stability.

## Fixing

- Once in a satisfactory position, ensure the lead and sheath are well sutured to the skin to minimize risk of displacement. Apply transparent occlusive dressings over the sheath and lead to help fix them in place and maintain sterility.
- Secure the external portion of the lead with tape or other fixatives.
- Fixing a loop on the skin should mean that inadvertent tugs on the wire will tighten the loop rather than pulling out the wire.

## Setting the box

- 'Output' should be set to three times the threshold, e.g. 3V.
- Set to 'demand' at a 'rate' of, for example, 70bpm.
- 'Demand' will mean it does not pace if intrinsic activity is sensed. Asynchronous pacing is therefore avoided and the risk of inducing ventricular arrhythmias reduced. The pacemaker will, on a beat-to-beat basis, 'pace' when it does not detect ventricular activity above that rate and the red 'pace' light will illuminate. When the spontaneous ventricular rate is above the pacemaker rate, the box will inhibit and the red 'sense' light will illuminate.
- 'Sensitivity' should be adjusted to ensure that each intrinsic beat is detected but that skeletal muscle interference does not lead to pacemaker inhibition (the lower the setting, the more sensitive the pacemaker 📖 p. 15).

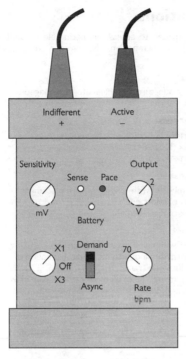

**Fig. 7.6** Temporary pacing box.

# Complications

These may be related to access, the pacing electrode, the connections, infections, or thromboembolism. The common complications depend on the access site.

### Jugular access

- Carotid artery puncture with haematoma managed with manual compression.

### Subclavian access

- Subclavian artery puncture with haemorrhage.
- Haemothorax (📖 p. 84).
- Pneumothorax (📖 p. 84).

### Femoral access

- Venous thrombosis (with long-term wire placement).
- Increased risk of infection.
- Increased risk of displacement.

### Pacing wire

- Dislodgement with failed pacing or intermittent pacing.
- Ventricular arrhythmia due to mechanical irritation of the RV.
- Fracture of electrode (rare).
- Perforation of myocardium with pericarditic pain, effusion, tamponade (📖 p .86).

# Other forms of temporary pacing

### Transcutaneous pacing

This technique is effective in up to 95% of cases but should be considered a temporary measure until a more definitive form of pacing therapy is available as it is uncomfortable for the conscious patient. Pads are placed in either an antero-posterior or antero-lateral arrangement. Alert patients are likely to require sedation and analgesia due to pectoral muscle contraction.

### Dual chamber temporary pacing

An additional atrial J preformed lead may be inserted from the subclavian or jugular approach. This may be required in patients dependent on A–V synchrony for satisfactory haemodynamics.

### Tunnelled temporary pacing system

This type of system is particularly useful in the pacing-dependent patient requiring explantation of an existing pacemaker system due to infection. A tunnelled single or dual chamber system may be implanted with the leads tunnelled on the front of the chest approximately 5cm from a subclavian or jugular point of access. These may be connected to a permanent pulse generator taped to the front of a chest and may remain in place for a number of weeks until the patient is ready for a new permanent system.

### Epicardial pacing

This is a common form of pacing post cardiac surgery with wires attached directly to the epicardium and passed through the skin (usually in the epigastric region). Although very useful in the immediate post-surgical phase, they suffer deterioration in performance and may become unusable by day 5–10.

### Transoesophageal pacing

This route has been proposed for emergency pacing in the conscious patient and requires an electrode to be passed via the oropharynx into the stomach with pacing through the diaphragm. It is rarely used because of the ease of transvenous pacing.

# Insertable loop recorder

# Introduction

Due to the episodic and infrequent nature of syncope, conventional investigation may fail to identify a cause in up to 70% of patients. Insertable loop recorders (ILR) provide extended rhythm monitoring for patients with syncope/presyncope in whom a diagnosis of cardiac arrhythmia is suspected.

At present the only commercially available ILR is the Medtronic Reveal device (XT and DX) (Fig. 8.1), which has the following characteristics:

• small: $61 \times 19 \times 8$mm; 8cm$^3$; 17g;
• bipolar electrode;
• 14 month battery life;
• solid state circular buffer: 21 minute memory;
• records subcutaneous ECG;
• graphical representation of heart rate data;
• patient activation;
• autoactivation by device;
• device interrogation using standard pacemaker equipment;
• cost approximately the same as that of a VVI pacemaker.

# Cost-effectiveness

In patients presenting with recurrent syncope the cost of an initial strategy of ILR implantation has been shown to compare favourably with that of an alternative strategy of electrophysiological study, external loop recorder, and tilt testing. The relevance of this analysis to clinical practice is not clear and, in general, ILRs are used in patients with recurrent syncope after other investigations have been negative.

Although not a complication of the device implantation itself, it is possible that a fatal arrhythmia may occur at the next recurrence of symptoms (rare with appropriate patient selection).

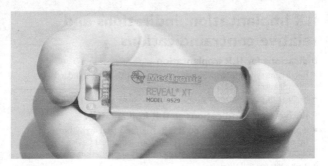

**Fig. 8.1** Insertable loop recorder (image reproduced with permission from Medtronic Inc).

# ILR implantation: indications and relative contraindications

### Indications for ILR implantation

- Recurrent syncope without definitive diagnosis after standard investigation.
- Recurrent presyncope without diagnosis after standard investigation.

### Relative contraindications to ILR implantation

- If patient is considered to be at high risk for a fatal arrhythmia on other grounds (e.g. low ejection fraction), empirical device therapy should be offered (e.g. ICD) instead of ILR implantation.
- Short life expectancy.
- Sepsis.
- Patient/carer unable to activate device (effectiveness therefore relies on autoactivation).

# ILR positioning

See Fig. 8.2.

- The technique for ILR implantation is essentially the same as that for inserting a pacemaker generator.
- Some centres implant ILRs in a ward/catheter laboratory setting but, ideally, a surgical theatre setting is preferable to minimize infection risks.
- It is recommended that the optimal location be identified using R-wave mapping prior to skin preparation (rarely done) by placing 2 ECG electrodes 4cm apart. The vector with the largest QRS complex is used to guide the position of the ILR.
- The standard placement is in the left midclavicular position between the 1st and 4th ribs.
- In young females the device may be placed in the left axillary position, which, in terms of R-wave sensed and arrhythmia sensed, can produce similar results to a parasternal position placement or via a submammary incision. The incision is made horizontally in the mid-axilla and the device implanted such that it avoids crossing the bra strap.

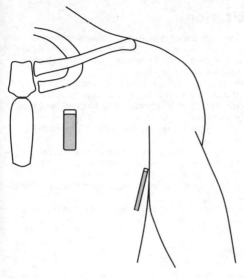

**Fig. 8.2** Positioning of ILR in the left parasternal and left axillary position.

# ILR implantation

- The skin is prepared and draped similarly to a pacemaker implant.
- For an axillary approach the patient can lift their left arm behind the head or be positioned on their right side with the left arm in front of the chest to expose the mid-axillary line.
- Infiltrate 10–20mL of 1% lignocaine at the incision site and pocket.
- A 2cm horizontal incision is made in the appropriate position.
- Fashion the pocket prepectorally (approximately 2 × 7cm) using blunt dissection and/or with dissecting scissors.
- The device is implanted and may be secured by a non-absorbable suture to the base of the pocket.
- Check the signal using a pacemaker wand in sterile plastic cover (assess presence of P waves and R wave amplitude).
- Reposition the device if parameters are not acceptable.
- Wound closed as for a pacemaker with subcutaneous and subcuticular sutures (📖 p. 68).
- The device is programmed and the patient/carer educated regarding the use of activator.

# Programming

ILRs require minimal programming. Memory can be frozen in response to patient activation, autoactivation, or both. Memory can be configured for patient activation or combined patient and autoactivation in a number of ways.

### Patient activation only
- 1 × activation (20min preactivation + 1min postactivation).
- 3 × activations (6 + 1min).

### Patient and autoactivation
- Heart rate < 40bpm for 4 consecutive beats: programmable to < 30bpm
- Heart rate > 165bpm: programmable to 115–230bpm. 16 or 32 consecutive beats.
- Asystole > 3.0s: programmable to > 4.0s.
- 1 × patient activation (6 + 1min) and 14 × autoactivation (1 + 1min).
- 3 × patient activation (4 + 1min) and 5 × autoactivation (1 + 1min).

# Complications

Complications following implantation of an ILR are rare. However, as with any implanted device the following may occur:
- pocket infection;
- erosion;
- migration.

## Pitfalls

- Poor ECG signal at implantation will limit the usefulness of any recordings, and may lead to inappropriate autoactivation.
- Failure to successfully activate the device after an event is common.
- MRI/radiofrequency fields/electrocautery may affect the programming of the ILR and cause spurious autodetections.
- Strong magnetic fields can attract the device, which may be uncomfortable for the patient.

# Diagnostic yield

This depends on the population studied, but reported overall yields are between 40% and 55%. The diagnostic yield is greater for patients with recurrent syncope (70%) versus presyncope (24%). An example of a positive finding from a Reveal implant is shown in Fig. 8.3.

# Interpretation: symptom–rhythm correlation

### Bradycardia
Detection of sudden onset of asystole/high degree AV block is an indication for permanent pacemaker implantation. However, amongst patients with recurrent syncope there is often a high incidence of neurocardiogenic syncope (📖 p. 40), comprising vasomotor and bradyarrhythmic components. Therefore a diagnosis of bradyarrhythmia does not necessarily mandate pacemaker implantation. Features to suggest neurocardiogenic syncope include:
- gradual onset of bradycardia, which may progress to AV block or asystole;
- oscillation of heart rate in sinus rhythm around the time of symptoms (often with a sinus acceleration before bradycardia).

**Tachyarrhythmia** Supraventricular or ventricular tachyarrhythmia correlating with symptoms should be managed along standard lines.

**Sinus rhythm** Demonstration of sinus rhythm during symptoms indicates a non-arrhythmic cause. Possibilities include predominantly vasomotor neurocardiogenic syncope, seizure (cyclical artefact on the recording may indicate seizure activity), or a psychological disorder.

# Explantation

At the end of life of the device (approximately 12–14 months) or when a definitive diagnosis has been made, the device may be explanted. This involves a simple removal under local anaesthesia through the original scar.

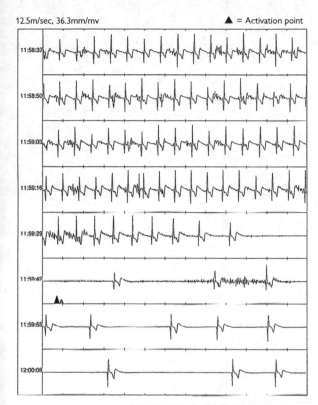

12.5m/sec, 36.3mm/mv                    ▲ = Activation point

**Fig. 8.3** Reveal recording. Data from a patient with recurrent syncope due to sinoatrial node disease and an 8s pause. Black triangle indicates time of patient activation.

# ICD principles

# Indications for ICD insertion

Historically (*circa* 1985), ICDs were reserved for individuals who had survived two prior cardiac arrests. At present, ICDs are also indicated for individuals identified as having a high risk of sudden cardiac death (SCD)—without the requirement for prior episodes of VT/VF.

## Clinical predictors of high arrhythmic death risk

These include:
- previous cardiac arrest due to VF, or haemodynamically poorly tolerated VT;
- previous sustained monomorphic VT;
- previous MI;
- coronary artery disease;
- heart failure: LVEF < 35%;
- prolonged QRS duration;
- genetic factors: HCM, long QT syndrome, Brugada syndrome, and arrhythmogenic right ventricular cardiomyopathy (ARVC).

## Problems with SCD risk stratification

- Highest risk groups (e.g. prior VF arrest) constitute the smallest proportion of the population at risk of SCD.
- 85–90% of SCD events are due to the first recognized arrhythmic event.
- Survival rates to hospital discharge for sudden cardiac arrest episodes are less than 5%.
- Non-invasive screening tests used in *individual* risk stratification have a low sensitivity (e.g. heart rate variability, Holter monitor, T-wave alternans, QT dispersion).

## Evidence base for ICD insertion

- Randomized trials sponsored by device companies.
- Historical meta-analyses of trials for 1° prevention (AVID, CASH, and CIDS) demonstrated benefit of ICDs over medical therapy (~ 50% reduction in risk of SCD).
- 1° prevention trials—heterogeneous designs make interpretation difficult. MADIT I and II, MUSTT, DEFINITE, COMPANION, and SCD HeFT demonstrate beneficial effects of ICDs on mortality. However, CABG Patch (post-CABG surgery) and DINAMIT (early post-MI) show no benefit.

# Clinical guidelines: introduction and NICE guidelines

There is a general consensus within Europe and the US regarding implantation of an ICD in survivors of a cardiac arrest, haemodynamically compromising VT, or VT on the background of severe LV impairment based on numerous studies (AVID, CIDS, CASH). However, in the primary implant setting, although the MADIT I data have been accepted and are routinely applied in both the US and Europe, there has been resistance (mainly on economic grounds) to undertake ICD implant for MADIT II grounds (EF < 30% and prior MI). The impact of implanting an ICD in all patients with an EF < 30% following an MI would be great and, unless the unit price for an ICD falls significantly, routine implantation on MADIT II grounds is unlikely to occur.

- In the UK, the NICE guidelines recommend implantation for MADIT II grounds **only** in patients with a broad QRS (>120ms) who are recognized to be a higher risk group than those with a narrow QRS.

## NICE guidelines[1]

An ICD is provided for a person who is in one of the following categories.
1 A person presents, in the absence of a treatable cause, with one of the following:
   - cardiac arrest due to either VT or VF; *or*
   - spontaneous sustained VT causing syncope or significant haemodynamic compromise; *or*
   - sustained VT without syncope or cardiac arrest, and who has an associated reduction in EF (LVEF < 35%) but is no worse than class III NYHA functional classification of heart failure.
2 A person has a history of an MI more than 4 weeks previously **and**
   - **either all** of the following:
     — left ventricular dysfunction with an LVEF of less than 35%, and no worse than class III NYHA functional classification of heart failure; *and*
     — non-sustained VT on Holter monitoring; *and*
     — inducible VT on EP testing.
   - **or both** of the following:
     — left ventricular dysfunction with an LVEF of less than 30% and no worse than class III NYHA functional classification of heart failure; *and*
     — QRS duration ≥ 120ms.
3 A person has a familial cardiac condition with a high risk of sudden death. (e.g. long QT syndrome, hypertrophic cardiomyopathy).
4 A person has undergone surgical repair of congenital heart disease.

## Technical points

- UK NICE guidelines do not include electrophysiological studies (EPS) in SCD risk stratification for patients with reduced LVEF presenting with unexplained syncope.
- US guidelines incorporate EPS for patients with MADIT I risk profiles, and for the investigation of syncope in patients with risk factors for SCD.

## Reference

1 National Institute for Health and Clinical Excellence (NICE) (1 January, 2006). *Implantable cardioverter defibrillators for arrhythmias, a review of the 2000 guidelines.* NICE, London.

# ACC/AHA/NASPE 2002 guidelines[2]

## Recommendations for ICD therapy

- Class I (good evidence).
  - Cardiac arrest due to VF or VT, not due to a transient or reversible cause (level of evidence: A).
  - Spontaneous sustained VT in association with structural heart disease (level of evidence: B).
  - Syncope of undetermined origin with clinically relevant, haemodynamically significant sustained VT or VF induced at EPS when drug therapy is ineffective, not tolerated, or not preferred (level of evidence: B).
  - Non-sustained VT in patients with coronary disease, prior MI, LV dysfunction, and inducible VF or sustained VT at EPS that is not suppressible by a class I anti-arrhythmic drug (level of evidence: A).
  - Spontaneous sustained VT in patients without structural heart disease, not amenable to other treatments (level of evidence: C).
- Class IIa (some evidence in favour).
  - Patients with LVEF ≤ 30% at least 1 month post-MI and 3 months post coronary artery revascularization surgery (level of evidence: B).
- Class IIb (some evidence in favour).
  - Cardiac arrest presumed to be due to VF when EPS is precluded by other medical conditions (level of evidence: C)
  - Severe symptoms (e.g. syncope) attributable to ventricular tachyarrhythmias in patients awaiting cardiac transplantation (level of evidence: C).
  - Familial or inherited conditions with a high risk for life-threatening ventricular tachyarrhythmias such as long QT syndrome or HCM (level of evidence: B).
  - Non-sustained VT with coronary artery disease, prior MI, LV dysfunction, and inducible sustained VT or VF at EPS (level of evidence: B)
  - Recurrent syncope of undetermined origin in the presence of ventricular dysfunction and inducible ventricular arrhythmias at EPS when other causes of syncope have been excluded (level of evidence: C).
  - Syncope of unexplained origin or family history of unexplained SCD in association with typical or atypical RBBB and ST-segment elevations (Brugada syndrome; level of evidence: C).
  - Syncope in patients with advanced structural heart disease in whom thorough invasive and non-invasive investigations have failed to define a cause (level of evidence: C).
- Class III.
  - Syncope of undetermined cause in a patient without inducible ventricular tachyarrhythmias and without structural heart disease (level of evidence: C).
  - Incessant VT or VF (level of evidence: C).

- VF or VT resulting from arrhythmias amenable to surgical or catheter ablation, e.g. atrial arrhythmias associated with the WPW syndrome, RVOT VT, idiopathic LV tachycardia, or fascicular VT (level of evidence: C).
- Ventricular tachyarrhythmia due to a transient or reversible disorder (e.g. AMI, electrolyte imbalance, drugs) when correction of the disorder is considered feasible and likely to substantially reduce the risk of recurrent arrhythmia (level of evidence: B).
- Significant psychiatric illnesses that may be aggravated by device implantation or may preclude systematic follow-up (level of evidence: C).
- Terminal illnesses with projected life expectancy < 6 months (level of evidence: C).
- Patients with coronary artery disease, LV dysfunction, and prolonged QRS duration in the absence of spontaneous or inducible sustained or non-sustained VT who are undergoing coronary bypass surgery (level of evidence: B).
- NYHA class IV drug-refractory CHF in patients who are not candidates for cardiac transplantation (level of evidence: C).

## Potential harms of ICD insertion

- Not recommended for patients in whom a reversible triggering factor for VT/VF can be definitively identified.
- Coronary disease patients without inducible or spontaneous VT undergoing routine coronary bypass surgery are not routine candidates for ICD therapy.
- Patients with WPW syndrome presenting with VF secondary to rapidly conducted AF should undergo ablation, if their accessory pathways are amenable to such treatment.
- Patients with terminal illness, NYHA class IV CHF who are not candidates for cardiac transplantation, or with a life expectancy not exceeding 6 months are likely to obtain limited benefit, if any, from ICD therapy. ICD implantation in such patients is discouraged.
- Psychiatric disorders, including uncontrolled depression and substance abuse that would interfere with the care and follow-up needed by these patients, are relative contraindications to device therapy.
- Patients with frequent tachyarrhythmias that may trigger shock therapy are not suitable candidates for an ICD. These events would cause frequent device activation and multiple shocks. Alternative therapies, such as combining drugs or ablation with ICD insertion, should be considered.

## Reference

2 ACC/AHA/NASPE (2002). ACC/AHA/NASPE 2002 guideline for implantation of cardiac pacemakers and antiarrhythmia devices: summary article. *J Cardiovasc Electrophysiol* **13**, 1200–1.

## How an ICD works

As originally devised by Michel Mirowski, the ICD was designed to provide electric shock therapy for ventricular tachyarrhythmias within a timeframe in which defibrillation efficacy approaches 100%. All devices have the following basic properties.

- Bradycardia pacing.
- Detection of ventricular arrhythmias.
- Discrimination of SVT, AF, sinus tachycardia.
- Tiered therapies based on ventricular rate or cycle length into maximum of three overlapping or non-overlapping zones (e.g. VT 150bpm or 400ms, fast VT 180bpm or 333ms, VF 240bpm or 250ms).
- Anti-tachycardia pacing (able to terminate 80% of monomorphic VT).
- Cardioversion and defibrillation for VT and VF (up to 41J output).
- Stored EGMs and marker recordings of events.
- Non-invasive electrophysiology testing.

# System elements

### Pulse generator (Fig. 9.1)

- Titanium casing: biologically inert, hermetically sealed.
- Lithium battery: ~ 3.2V at full charge with approximately 5 year lifespan.
- Capacitors: charged via battery and DC-DC converters to store 30–41J within 10–30s. Deliver up to 750V defibrillation energy over 10–20ms.
- Microprocessor: programmable detection algorithms permit tailored therapies, stored diagnostics for device interrogation, and PES.
- Telemetry communication coil: for all non-invasive programming.
- Size: approximately 70–85g weight and 30–40cm$^3$ volume.
- Aerial: new devices may have wireless communication between the ICD and programmer.
- 'Hot can': generator also acts as an electrode in shock circuit therefore allowing different defibrillation vectors by employing different combinations of shock electrodes. All modern devices now incorporate the can as an electrode.
- Ventricular sensing: always bipolar but may be true bipolar (tip to proximal ring electrode) or integrated bipolar (tip to distal RV shock electrode).

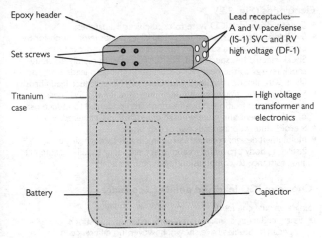

**Fig. 9.1** Schematic diagram showing features of a dual chamber ICD.

### Electrodes (Fig. 9.2)

- Endocardial: older ICD systems used epicardial patches.
- Single/dual chamber: an additional atrial lead adds information for SVT discrimination and also allows for dual chamber bradycardia pacing.
- Shock electrodes: specialized, high surface area to rapidly distribute shock energy to the heart for defibrillation (modern leads are back filled with silicone or coated with Gore ePTFE to reduce lead fibrosis).
- Single/dual coil: single coil RV only; dual have RV and SVC coils.
- Active/passive fixation: active fixation often preferred to reduce risk of dislodgement and increase ease of extraction if required.
- Steroid eluting tip: reduces risk of exit block.
- Multilumen design: conductors run in parallel through single insulating body providing greater space efficiency (smaller diameter) and resistance to compression (previously coaxial).

#### Choice of ICD lead and points to consider

##### Single or dual coil lead?

- Single coil leads are associated with an increase in shock impedance. Studies have shown, however, no difference in defibrillation threshold (DFT) between dual coil and single coil.
- In individual patients, using an RV coil only may significantly reduce the DFT and the opposite is also true. It is, however, easier to remove the SVC coil either electronically or manually (by removing the DF-1 pin from the port on the ICD) than to add a separate SVC coil or change to a new dual coil lead.
- The additional SVC coil on a dual coil lead can lead to intense fibrous adhesion that can make lead extraction in the future very difficult.

##### Active or passive fixation?

- Active fixation allows for positioning of the V lead in positions other than the apex where a passive lead would be stable. Active leads are also easier to extract as the active fixation mechanism can be undone and there are no tines present.
- Active fixation can rarely lead to perforation of the myocardium, pericarditis, effusion, and, rarely, tamponade.

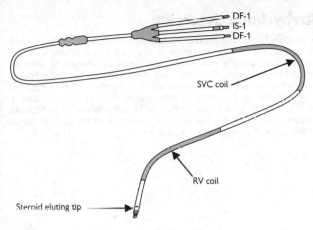

DF-1
IS-1
DF-1

SVC coil

RV coil

Steroid eluting tip

**Fig. 9.2** Schematic diagram of a dual coil active ICD lead.

## Arrhythmia detection

In both single and dual chamber devices a hierarchical set of criteria need to be met in order for the device to diagnose an arrhythmia. The first and most important is ventricular rate. In order to differentiate ventricular arrhythmias from SVTs, AF, and sinus tachycardia, discriminators (which are present on both single and dual chamber devices) are used (Fig. 9.3). With dual chamber devices, information is also taken from the atrial channel to again decide on the type of tachycardia in order to avoid inappropriate therapies. The effect of premature ventricular stimulation (PVS) on the rhythm can also be assessed.

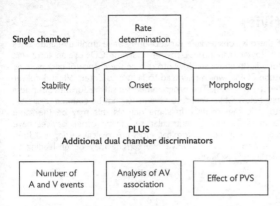

**Fig. 9.3** Generic single and dual chamber SVT discrimination.

# Sensitivity

During VF there is considerable variation in R-wave amplitude and values are normally lower than intrinsic rhythm. Current ICDs use an automatic beat-to-beat adjustment of sensitivity to reduce the chance of undersensing low amplitude EGMs, which may lead to failure to detect VF and deliver prompt therapy (Fig. 9.4). The programmed sensitivity for an ICD refers to the setting below which ventricular events will not be counted regardless of the automatic gain control. In some devices this may be the same value as bradycardia pacing ventricular sensitivity; other devices have standard settings (e.g. 'Least, Nominal, Most'). A typical setting is 0.3mV. If a device is too sensitive T-wave oversensing may occur leading to double counting (📖 p. 258).

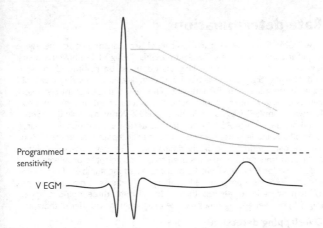

**Fig. 9.4** Ventricular EGM during sinus rhythm with automatic adjustment of sensitivity. Three different examples are shown. Sensing starts at a percentage (50–80%) of the sensed R wave and then decays linearly, exponentially, or initially constant and then a linear decay. This allows for sensing of low amplitude VF and avoids T-wave oversensing. With a paced event similar adjustment occurs after the blanking period. Different parameters can be programmed depending on the device. The dotted line represents the programmed sensitivity below which events will be ignored.

# Rate determination

Raw EGMs from the ventricular channel are transmitted to the sense amplifier and then filtered. Fibrillation EGMs during VF are high frequency low amplitude events so blanking periods must be minimized to avoid undersensing. Signals are rectified and compared to a sensing threshold to generate a series of RR intervals. The device must accurately detect events over a wide range of amplitudes (paced event 5000mV; intrinsic R wave ~ 10mV; PVCs and VT 5–25mV; VF 0.2–20mV; asystole 0–0.15mV). Fixed sensing thresholds do not permit accurate transition from large to small amplitude sensed events without unacceptable errors (e.g. P- or T-wave oversensing, lack of discrimination of VF from asystole). Automatic adjustment of sensitivity is used to overcome these problems.

An episode of VT or VF will be declared when the number of ventricular episodes exceeds a programmed level, e.g. 12/16 beats at rate greater than 170bpm or cycle length less than 353ms. Up to three non-overlapping (Fig. 9.5) or overlapping zones may be programmed with tiered therapies.

## Overlapping detection

Some devices allow for overlapping detection zones. Commonly the FVT zone can be programmed to detect 'via VF'. In Fig. 9.6 the device has been programmed such that VF detection requires 18/24 R–R intervals to have a rate > 188bpm. When any of the final eight R–R intervals preceding the moment of detection has a rate > 240bpm (cycle length < 250ms) the episode is classified as VF. If all of the last eight R–R intervals have a rate < 240bpm it is classified as FVT. A rate of > 240bpm is classified as VF.

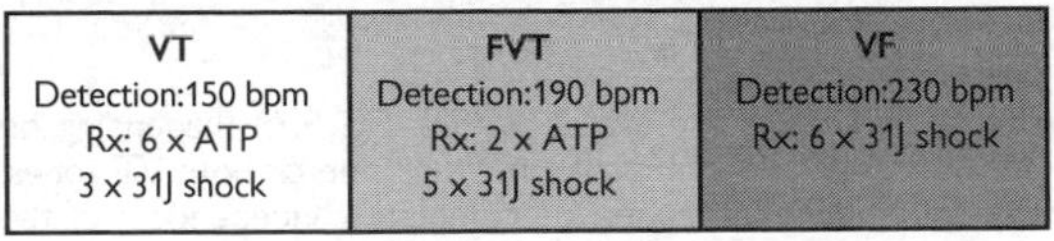

VT
Detection:150 bpm
Rx: 6 x ATP
3 x 31J shock
FVT
Detection:190 bpm
Rx: 2 x ATP
5 x 31J shock
VF
Detection:230 bpm
Rx: 6 x 31J shock

**Fig. 9.5** Example of three non-overlapping detection zones. Note that no ATP is programmable in the VF zone.

167
VT
188
188
FVT
240
188
VF
500

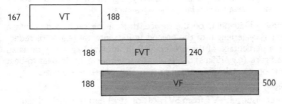

**Fig. 9.6** FVT via VF. Ventricular rates in bpm.

# SVT discriminators

The following discriminators are available. (See Fig. 9.7.) Depending on the device these may be programmable in either one or both VT zones, independently within both VT zones, or completely independent of the VT and VF zones.

## Sudden onset of ventricular rate

A programmable 'sudden onset' was designed to avoid inappropriate therapies for sinus tachycardia. It is very specific for the rejection of sinus tachycardia but can have a low sensitivity, e.g. when VT occurs during exercise with only a small relative increase in rate.

*Programming* Depending on the device, this can be set as a percentage reduction in cycle length of the preceding R–R interval (e.g. a 9% reduction), or a percentage of the preceding R–R interval (e.g. 84%), or as an absolute figure (e.g. 150ms). Algorithms use either a single beat-to-beat R–R value or may take an average of a number of preceding beats.

*Problems*
- It cannot distinguish VT from SVT, AF, or atrial flutter, which all can have a sudden onset.
- In cases of slow VT below the detection rate for VT this may then accelerate into the VT zone and sudden onset criteria will not be met.
- Slow VTs may have gradual accelerations and decelerations and may cross into and out of the detection zones.

## Ventricular stability

'Stability' was designed to detect episodes of AF where the R–R interval is generally irregular. It is highly specific for the rejection of relatively slow AF, which are usually below the detection zone. The R–R interval is compared to either a mean of a number of R–R intervals or a reference updated during the tachycardia.

*Programming* This is programmed as an absolute figure (e.g. 40ms). In some devices the number of intervals or time over which stability is assessed is programmable.

*Problems*
- Monomorphic VT may be unstable especially in the presence of anti-arrhythmic agents or when the rate is slow.
- Atrial fibrillation with high ventricular rates (> 170bpm) can appear to be relatively stable, i.e. the range of irregularity is less than 40ms.
- Polymorphic VT will be unstable but usually falls in the VF zone where SVT discriminators do not operate.

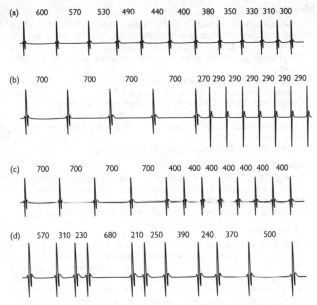

**Fig. 9.7** Ventricular EGMs demonstrating use and difficulties of sudden onset and stability as SVT discriminators. (a) Sinus tachycardia. There is a gradual decrease in the R–R interval with no sudden onset. (b) Ventricular tachycardia. There is a sudden onset of shortening of R–R interval. The cycle length in VT is stable. Note also the change in EGM morphology compared to the preceding sinus beats. (c) Atrial flutter. There is a sudden shortening of R–R interval, the EGM morphology staying unchanged throughout. The cycle length is stable. (d) AF. The cycle length is unstable throughout.

## Morphology

The morphology of any bipolar EGM is determined by the vector (direction) of local depolarization at the electrode tip. This vector changes with bundle branch block, rate-dependent aberrancy, and VT.

Morphology algorithms in modern devices work using the following method.

- Obtain a template EGM *during sinus rhythm*.
- Template is updated at regular intervals, e.g. daily.
- Compare the EGM of the tachycardia beats to the template.
- A defined number of tachycardia beats needs to have a specific percentage match to the template (e.g. 5 of 8 beats ≥ 60% match) to be labelled as SVT.
- In some devices these parameters are programmable.

### Problems

- If morphology is the only discriminator in a single chamber device, rate-related bundle branch block during sinus tachycardia or atrial fibrillation will be labelled as VT.
- Cannot be used in patients with intermittent bundle branch block.

## SVT override

Most devices have a feature that overrides SVT discriminators after a programmable period ('sustained rate duration', 'high rate timeout', 'maximum time to diagnosis'). These discriminators were designed to protect against inappropriate withholding of therapy for prolonged episode of VT. However they do increase the risk of inappropriate therapies for SVTs. If programmed 'on', any episode fulfilling the rate criteria for VT will have therapy delivered after the programmed period even if all of the SVT criteria are satisfied.

**Problem** Sustained SVT for longer than the programmed period will be inappropriately treated as VT.

# Dual chamber SVT discriminators

The method of discriminating SVT from VT in dual chamber devices is based on the method in single chamber devices with the additional information from the atrial channel (Fig. 9.8).

It is important to remember that a number of potential A:V relationships are possible during ventricular arrhythmias:

- V > A (VA dissociation with VT);
- A > V (VT with AF);
- V = A (VT with retrograde 1:1 VA conduction).

Due to these possible associations during ventricular arrhythmias, dual chamber algorithms were developed. The combination of discriminators used varies between manufactures but is generally divided into three arms dependent on the A:V association.

### Medtronic enhanced PR logic and wavelet dynamic discrimination

Wavelet dynamic discrimination is based on wavelet decomposition of EGMs from six different configuration of near- and far-field EGMs (commonly RV coil-can is used as appears to be less affected by increase in heart rate during exercise). A nominal match threshold of 70% is used compared to the sinus template.

Enhanced PR logic analyses A–V associations assuming that tachycardias fit similar patterns. It analyses the V–V intervals of each ventricular event and assigns a code depending on the position and number of atrial events within these intervals and the zone in which those atrial events occur. This code is then compared to stored tachyarrhythmia codes to classify the event and decide if therapy is appropriate.

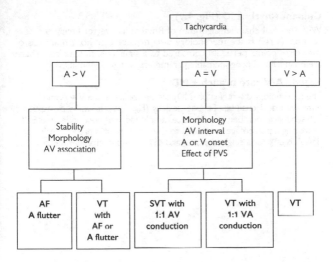

**Fig. 9.8** Dual chamber SVT discrimination. The initial requirement in declaring an episode is the ventricular rate. When the rate is sufficient, in a dual chamber device, three limbs of discrimination are available. If atrial rate is greater than ventricular rate, stability, morphology, and AV association can be used to discriminate between an atrial and ventricular rates are the same, morphology, the A–V interval, the effect of premature ventricular stimulation (PVS), and whether the arrhythmia started in the atrium or ventricle can be used. These try to discriminate an SVT with 1:1 conduction from VT with 1:1 retrograde VA conduction. If the ventricular rate is greater than atrial the episode is VT.

### Guidant Rhythm ID (Fig. 9.9)

With the dual chamber algorithm of Rhythm ID, 'vector timing and correlation' (VTC) is the morphology discriminator based on an analysis of over eight points per EGM compared to a sinus rhythm template. There are no individual programmable parameters within Rhythm ID.

### St Jude A/V rate branch + MD

The morphology discriminator (MD) can be applied in the V = A and V < A arms with dual chamber St Jude devices (Fig. 9.10). It works by assessing the sequence, number, polarity, size, amplitude, and area under the EGM producing a percentage compared to the template. It is programmable and default is 60% for a single chamber and 45% for a dual chamber device.

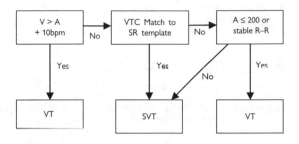

**Fig. 9.9** Rhythm ID.

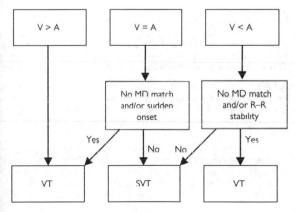

**Fig. 9.10** A/V rate branch + MD.

## Tachyarrhythmia therapies

Programming should be patient-specific and balanced between early defibrillation for highest risk arrhythmias and attempts at ATP for non-life-threatening arrhythmias at rates not likely to result in syncope. Tiered therapy is available:
- anti-tachycardia pacing (ATP);
- cardioversion;
- defibrillation.

## Anti-tachycardia pacing

ATP is designed to interrupt re-entrant VT circuits using pacing-level stimuli at maximum output that is well tolerated by patients (often asymptomatic or detected as 'palpitations'). It is utilized in the FVT and VT zones and some modern devices can deliver ATP whilst charging for cardioversion.
- Highly effective at terminating spontaneous VT (approximately 90%).
- Reduces the frequency of ICD defibrillation therapies.
- 1–5% risk of accelerating arrhythmia.
- Programmed to pace at an R–R interval as percentage of the cycle length of the VT (e.g. 84%) to maximize chance of capture.

### Redetection

The device monitors for an outcome following each ATP therapy cycle. If the device redetects the original arrhythmia after an ATP sequence, it delivers the next ATP sequence. If the tachycardia accelerates into a faster zone, the remaining sequences of ATP are not delivered and the device delivers the next programmed therapy for the new zone.

### Types of ATP

*Burst (Fig. 9.11)* Fixed R–R interval between delivered pulses in a sequence. The pacing interval for the first burst sequence is calculated as a programmable percentage of the tachycardia cycle length. Therapy is delivered in VOO mode.

*Ramp (Fig. 9.12)* As for burst pacing, the first pulse of each ramp sequence is delivered at a calculated percentage of the current tachycardia cycle length. However, each remaining pulse in that sequence is then delivered at progressively shorter intervals by subtracting, per pulse, the programmed interval decrement to a programmed minimal interval (usually 200ms). Therapy is delivered in VVI mode (sensed events are counted as individual pulses of the ramp sequence).

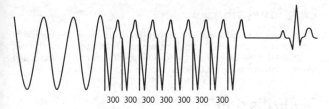

**Fig. 9.11** Burst ATP with intervals in ms.

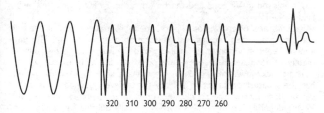

**Fig. 9.12** Ramp ATP with intervals in ms.

## Failure of ATP

Following failure of ATP to terminate VT and redetection of this, there are a number of programmable features to make the next ATP more aggressive.
- Addition of one or more pulses to each successive ATP burst.
- Reassessment of the VT rate before further burst in case VT has accelerated but remained within the same VT zone.
- Incrementally reduce the pacing cycle length after each ATP burst.

# Cardioversion

This is a synchronized shock to a sensed ventricular event (the key difference from a defibrillation shock). Devices can cardiovert at up to 41J from the device and this may be used in the FVT and VT zones. The vector and programming are as for defibrillation shocks.

# Defibrillation

Defibrillation requires depolarization of the majority of the ventricular myocardium and this may require up to 41J DC shock. It is the **only** therapy employed in VF zone and can be utilized in FVT/VT zones following failure of ATP.

Patients are often syncopal prior to appropriate defibrillations and consciousness often returns with restoration of sinus rhythm. The time interval between VF onset and delivery of defibrillation therapy is approximately 10–15s (capacitor charge time principally accounts for delay).

The shock waveform (Fig. 9.13) is a biphasic shock waveform and this has the greatest defibrillation efficacy for transvenous leads. The shock vector depends on the shock electrodes utilized: programmable, with lowest defibrillation thresholds (DFTs) typically utilizing RV apical shock electrode as anode and involving ICD shell ('hot can') in the circuit in left-sided pectoral systems. There are a number of parameters regarding detection and pacing around the time of defibrillation.

- Confirming VF after initial detection. May be programmed to 'yes' before first therapy to prevent committed therapies in the context of non-sustained ventricular arrhythmias. Reconfirmation of VF does not apply for subsequent therapies for a particular episode in order to reduce the delay to defibrillation in refractory VF.
- VT detection following defibrillation. Suspended to avoid detecting transient VT that may follow high voltage therapies.
- Post-shock pacing. Output increased transiently to ensure capture following successful defibrillation.

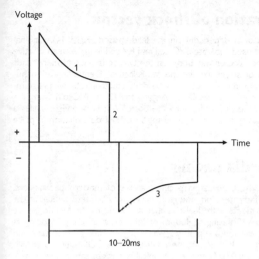

**Fig. 9.13** Biphasic defibrillation pulse waveform. (1) Decay truncated typically after ~ 50% decay. (2) Reversal of remaining voltage polarity over 2–3ms. (3) Second segment of waveform truncated after ~ 50% decay. Some new devices allow for programming of the waveform in terms of pulse width, polarity, and tilt.

## Configuration of shock vector

The shock vector is dependent on the lead(s) used (Fig. 9.14). Original venous systems used separate SVC coil and RV coil leads with an inactive can so the shock vector was between the two coils only. Modern leads are either dual or single soil and the can is 'active'. Depending on manufacturer, removing the SVC coil may be done electronically via programming or may require physically unplugging the DF-1 SVC pin from the device and insertion of a plug into the port. With very difficult cases a subcutaneous array may be required for successful defibrillation in place of the SVC coil.

## Bradycardia pacing

ICDs have all the bradycardia pacing features of modern pacemakers. Unless clearly indicated, 'physiological' pacing may be detrimental. In the DAVID trial, patients with dual chamber ICDs and LV dysfunction were randomized to VVI pacing at 40bpm or 'physiological' DDDR pacing at 70bpm. At 1-year follow-up there was a higher rate of mortality and congestive heart failure (CHF) hospitalizations in DDDR group (83.9% versus 73.3%, $p = 0.03$). Therefore RV apical pacing appears detrimental—probably due to induced intra- and interventricular dyssynchrony.

Programmable post-shock pacing parameters are available to prevent pauses post-shock. These may be programmed separately from the bradycardia pacing or may need to be programmed the same as for the bradycardia pacing. During post-shock pacing higher outputs are required to account for shock-induced increases in pacing thresholds.

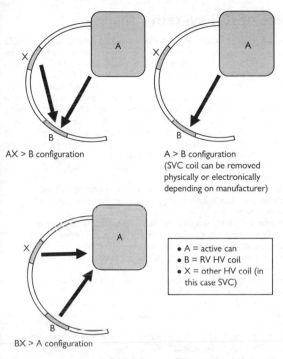

AX > B configuration

A > B configuration
(SVC coil can be removed
physically or electronically
depending on manufacturer)

BX > A configuration

- A = active can
- B = RV HV coil
- X = other HV coil (in
  this case SVC)

**Fig. 9.14** Shock vector configuration.

# Choice of ICD system

As opposed to pacemakers, when considering what type of leads and ICD to implant it is important to consider the implications of multiple large leads and the future need of extraction. Atrial leads have now been shown to reduce inappropriate therapies by improving SVT discrimination. However, they reduce battery longevity (approximately 4.7 years for single versus 4.0 years for dual lead systems—varies between manufacturers) and increase the need for re-operation due to atrial lead dislodgement. Approximately 10% of patients who receive ICDs for secondary prevention have a primary indication for bradycardia pacing at initial implant, and approximately 30% have class II indications. It is therefore important to consider all factors when making the decision.

The following considerations are important when considering single versus dual chamber.
- Bradycardia-related indication for dual chamber pacing: patients with complete heart block, sinoatrial node disease should receive dual chamber device.
- Permanent AF: all patients should receive single chamber device.
- Patient age: young patients have greater lifetime risk of lead-related complications (single lead systems are easier to extract).
- Known paroxysmal AF and SVT: an additional atrial lead will improve discrimination of SVT.
- LV function and NYHA class: patients with symptomatic impaired LV function may be a candidate for a CRT-D (📖 p. 276).
- Non-bradycardia related indications for dual chamber pacing:
  - patients with obstructive HCM requiring RV apical pacing to reduce LVOT gradient;
  - congenital long QT syndrome patients requiring high base-rate pacing to reduce the risk of PVCs and short–long sequences, leading to torsades de pointes polymorphic VT.

# ICD implantation

# Pre-procedure assessment

The basic operative technique shares many features with permanent pacemaker insertion (📖 p. 52). Those factors unique to ICD implantation will be covered here.

## Pre-operative evaluation

- Appropriateness of ICD therapy. Confirm that it fulfils current guidelines (📖 pp. 190–3).
- Fitness for procedure. Exclude infection and absence of uncontrolled CHF symptoms.
- Cardiac anatomy. Particular note should be made of evidence of prior inferior MI; suggests R-wave amplitude may be poor with preferred RV apical ICD lead placement.
- Baseline rhythm. Ideally with Holter monitoring, to identify paroxysmal SVTs (especially PAF), which may affect type of device implanted.
- Medications: warfarin (stop prior to operation, ± heparin cover), amiodarone (may increase DFTs).
- Decision on general anaesthetic (GA) or sedation. Although an ICD implant can be performed comfortably under sedation and local anaesthesia, DFTs require deeper sedation (e.g. midazolam plus fentanyl) or GA. The decision on which to use will depend on the patient's clinical status, preference, and local policy.

## Counselling and consent

Patients need to be fully aware of the benefits but also the downsides to ICD implantation as well as lifestyle implications.

- Acute operative risks. ~ 5% major complication rate (e.g. cardiac tamponade, pneumothorax, haemothorax, haematoma, arrhythmia with lead placement).
- 30 day mortality. ~ 3% from historical 2° prevention trials (no different from medically treated patients). More recent data (COMPANION trial) for 1° prevention of SCD with CRT–ICD implantation demonstrated a 0.5–0.8% operative mortality and 1.0–1.8% 30-day mortality.
- Chronic complications include: infection (requiring system extraction, ~ 0.5–1.0%); lead displacement (~ 4% for atrial, < 1% for ventricular); venous thrombosis (rarely symptomatic).
- Inappropriate ICD discharge rate. Estimates vary: ~ 2.5%/year from SCD HeFT trial. This is an important consideration as an inappropriate shock will usually occur with the patient conscious and therefore can be very uncomfortable,
- Proarrhythmia. Small risk from ATP (VT accelerated, causing syncope) but defibrillation shock available as rescue therapy.
- Driving restrictions. In the UK the patient will not be able to drive for 1 month after a primary implant and 6 months after a secondary prevention implant. Patients will not be able to drive for 6 months after an appropriate shock (📖 p. 346).

## Medications

### *Warfarin*
If warfarin is stopped in a patient with atrial fibrillation, DFTs should be avoided due to the risk of thromboembolism.

### *Amiodarone*
With modern biphasic waveforms, amiodarone use is associated with a small increase in defibrillation threshold (approx. 1.5J).

### *Beta-blockers*
These produce a small reduction in defibrillation thresholds (approx. 1.5J).

### *Sotalol*
Animal studies have previously shown sotalol to reduce defibrillation threshold significantly. More recent human studies have shown a small reduction in threshold similar to conventional beta-blockers without class III action.

# Patient and equipment preparation

## Patient preparation

- IV antibiotics. A combination of benzylpenicillin and flucloxacillin, or vancomycin if penicillin-allergic, to reduce the risk of device infection (see local policy regarding prophylactic antibiotics).
- Anxiolytic: optional.
- IV access on ipsilateral side to the device. Venography may be required for axillary or subclavian vein puncture.

## Equipment and staff

- Device-specific programmer.
  - Wand and sterile sleeve.
- Pacing system analyser (PSA).
  - As per bradycardia implants. Measures pacing thresholds and impedances.
- External defibrillator. Attach pads prior to draping patient.
- ICD and leads.
  - Turn tachycardia therapies off prior to implant.
  - Check battery voltage. 3.2V (beginning of life indicator; BOL) and perform capacitor maintenance charge (should be < 15s at BOL).
  - Have backup device (and any other sterile equipment) available.
- Personnel.
  - Nurses: scrub and circulating nurse.
  - ICD technician ± device manufacturer technical support.
  - Radiographer (in some departments).
  - Anaesthetist/sedating physician or nurse.

## Sedation versus general anaesthetic

This needs to be discussed prior to the procedure. Points to consider include:

- patient preference;
- type of pocket (submuscular pocket is more painful);
- age and co-morbidity of patient.

# Implant procedure

The left side is used preferentially due to a lower DFT (unless contraindication such as previous trauma, infection or scarring).

## Skin preparation, pocket fashioning, and venous access

- Drape and prepare the skin as for a pacemaker; infiltrate local anaesthesia.
- Make either a subcutaneous or submuscular pocket (depending on the amount of tissue present; 📖 p. 54). The pocket needs to be significantly larger compared to that for a pacemaker.
- Obtain venous access (cephalic or axillary vein preferred—minimizes risk of subclavian crush and pneumothorax although physician preference also plays a role; 📖 p. 56).

## Lead placement

- Place the ventricular ICD lead (some operators advocate active leads for all patients) in the RV apex (associated with lowest DFTs).
- Accept an R wave > 5mV (ensures < 10% undersensing during VF). If an acceptable R wave and threshold cannot be found then try other positions (active lead increases the flexibility of positions that can be tried) including the interventricular septum and RVOT.
- The ICD lead impedance is 300–1500 ohms, depending upon lead type.
- Place the atrial lead. Some operators prefer straight atrial lead with J-shaped stylets as it permits more lateral placement than pre-formed J-shaped lead, when usual atrial appendage position results in unacceptable parameters.
- Accept a P wave > 2mV.
- Accept pacing thresholds < 1V at 0.5ms.
- Once acceptable parameters are obtained secure the leads as for pacing leads with non-absorbable material (e.g. silk).

## Device connection and implant

- Connect the device to the leads making sure that the correct pins go into each receptacle.
- If a single coil ICD lead is used then a commercially available plug should be put into the SVC coil port of the ICD.
- Once connected implant the device into the pocket, making sure there is adequate room in the pocket to allow for good wound closure.

# Device testing

Test the device prior to closing the pocket as this permits lead repositioning if any parameters are inadequate. Use a sterile cover over the
programming wand and place the wand over the device.

### Pacing parameters
- Re-check pacing thresholds and impedances (□ p. 66).
- Ensure adequate EGMs. Make sure there is no noise on the EGMs
  indicating either a defective or damaged lead or possibly a poor
  connection on the header.
- Leads should be repositioned at this stage if there is any concern.

### High voltage (HV) lead integrity check
- Ensure the patient is adequately sedated.
- Deliver 12V synchronous stimulus through coils (< 1J).
- Assess the shock impedance: normal range ~ 30–70 ohms.
  - > 100 ohms suggests either pins not secure in header, or
    conductor/shocking coil fracture.
  - < 30 ohms suggests possible insulation breech.

# DFTs and atrial fibrillation

Patients with chronic AF undergoing ICD implantation should be treated
as though they are undergoing cardioversion as DFT may result in sinus
rhythm. Therefore patients should receive anticoagulation for 4 weeks
prior if possible. Patients may present with an indication for an ICD and
asymptomatic AF that has not been noted before. In this case transoesophageal echocardiography to exclude left atrial appendage thrombus
may be performed and the patient anticoagulated.

# Defibrillation threshold testing

Prior to performing DFTs ensure all personnel are ready and patient adequately sedated. One qualified member of staff should man the external defibrillator during the testing. Testing aims to check the worst case scenario, i.e. VF rather than VT, and at the least sensitive setting with the aim of having a 10J safety margin (i.e. testing successfully at 10J less than the maximum output of the device).

- Programme the ICD.
  - Programme a single VF zone only at 188bpm.
  - Programme sensitivity to least sensitive setting.
  - Programme a 1st shock at 10J below maximum output and a 2nd shock at maximum output (e.g. 25J, then 35J).
- Turn on real time printer prior to induction.
- Induction of VF (Fig. 10.1) can be performed by:
  - drive train of eight paced beats followed by low output shock (e.g. 1–1.5J) timed to the peak of the T wave on the surface ECG (if unsuccessful confirm timing of shock);
  - short burst of 50Hz pacing (2–4s);
  - direct current fibrillator;
  - alternating current (can be painful due to skeletal muscle stimulation).
- If the two shocks from the device fail to successfully defibrillate the patient deliver an external 'rescue' defibrillation at maximum output.
- If this fails to defibrillate the patient, commence CPR and attempt simultaneous external defibrillation with a commanded maximum output shock from the device.

Following successful defibrillation:
- Review the following.
  - Sensing EGMs (acceptable VF sensing < 10% 'drop-out').
  - Charge time.
  - Shock impedance.
  - Re-check lead position (may be dislodged following defibrillation).
- Wait at least 5min between inductions to avoid iatrogenic high DFT in the immediate post-shock period.
- Repeat for second DFT (some operators perform only one implant with a 10J safety margin for primary prevention implants).
- Pocket closure.
  - Device tachycardia therapies turned off during closure.
  - Gentamicin 80mg often given into pocket.

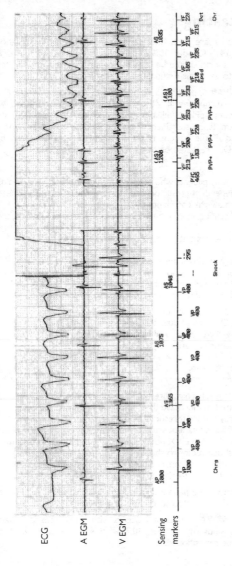

**Fig. 10.1** Successful induction of VF using 'Shock on T'. Eight paced beats (VP) at CL 400ms followed by shock after final paced beat. Excellent sensing in the VF zone.

# Difficult testing

Most ICD implants are straightforward and successful defibrillation thresholds (< 20J) are found in 90% of patients using a single coil lead. A maximum of 4–5 shocks should be used during any one test as repeated shocks may lead to ventricular stunning and heart failure.

**Unable to induce** It is sometimes impossible to induce VF despite using all available techniques. If VT occurs below the programmed VF zone then 50Hz burst applied whilst in VT may convert the rhythm to VF. If, despite all attempts, no sustained VF can be induced testing may have to be abandoned. If the patient is on anti-arrhythmics, these can be stopped and the DFT repeated off this a number of weeks later.

## High DFT

It is difficult to identify patients who will have high defibrillation thresholds. The only two independent predictors are LV mass and a fast resting heart rate (but only with a weak correlation).

If, despite good sensing, there is a high defibrillation threshold first exclude reversible causes:
• high voltage connections at header not complete (high shock impedance);
• pneumothorax (high shock impedance, hypoxia);
• hypoxia (low oxygen saturation);
• myocardial ischaemia (examine the ECG);
• poor lead position or dislodgement (fluoroscopy).

Having excluded these, the options include:
• removal of the SVC coil (if dual coil used);
• if a single coil lead change to dual coil lead (occasionally successful);
• reversal of the shock polarity;
• optimization of the defibrillation waveform (St Jude only);
• repositioning of the lead;
• changing device to high energy device (e.g. from 31J to 41J maximum).

If despite this there is still a high threshold the options include the following:
• stop amiodarone (may increase threshold) and retest later.
• start sotalol (may reduce threshold) and retest later.
• implantation of a subcutaneous array (tunnelled in the left lateral chest tissue, connected to the HVX port usually occupied by SVC coil pin) to change the shock vector to shunt more current through the LV.
• inserting a coil into the coronary sinus (there are case reports demonstrating a benefit) to change the shock vector.

The decision whether the patient should remain an inpatient for further testing will depend on the clinical scenario (e.g. primary prevention).

**Undersensing of VF** This usually occurs with a low sensed R-wave amplitude during sinus rhythm (Fig. 10.2). If this is the case, the lead usually needs to be repositioned.

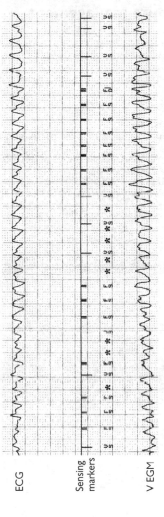

**Fig. 10.2** Undersensing of VF. Multiple R waves during VF are not sensed (*). Due to the undersensing many events are misclassified as sinus beats (VS). Eventually VF is detected (FD) but immediately to lowering detection further undersensing leads to classification of events as sinus (VS).

# Post-procedure management

- Programme device detection and therapies 'on'.
- Ensure sensitivity is reprogrammed to 'nominal' (e.g. 0.3mV).
- Print and review settings prior to leaving theatre and save settings to disk.
- CXR: check for lead positioning and exclude pneumothorax.
- ECG.
- IV antibiotics: one or two further doses (if complicated procedure or re-do, a 3–5 day course may be prescribed).
- Overnight cardiac monitor.
- ICD interrogation: next day, prior to discharge to confirm stable lead parameters.
- Some units perform further DFTs the day following implant.
- Follow-up and discharge instructions:
  - follow-up usually in 4–6 weeks in ICD clinic;
  - provide contact numbers in case of problems (e.g. ICD therapies, wound concerns);
  - provide device identification card;
  - non-absorbable suture removal in 7–10 days;
  - advise of driving regulations (📖 p. 346).

## Alternative methods of defibrillation testing

- Step down to failure, e.g. sequentially 36J, 30J, 25J until fails to defibrillate.
- Step down to failure with repeat testing (as above but repeat testing at lowest successful output).
- Upper limit of vulnerability (alternative method used for research purposes involving low output shocks in vulnerable periods as a marker of defibrillation threshold).

These techniques have been previously used for testing. It is increasingly recommended to reduce the number of shocks a patient receives, especially with the advent of active cans, smaller devices, and higher outputs.

# ICD programming

# Introduction

Programming is often performed on an individual patient basis, tailoring therapies and detection criteria to clinical history and documented arrhythmias. There is no evidence, however, that this strategy improves outcome or reduces the morbidity associated with inappropriate shocks. Recent studies have demonstrated that empirical programming (EMPIRIC PainFREE Rx II) may be as good as tailored therapy. However, information obtained during patient follow-up will allow for fine tuning of device programming. Although many devices are implanted for VF arrests, it is important to remember that the most common tachyarrhythmia detected by ICDs is VT and VF is often preceded by VT.

# Detection zones and therapies

Although there is no evidence that empirical programming of ICDs is any worse than tailored programming, there are some important points to note. Detection zones can be programmed in 1–3 non-overlapping or, in some devices, overlapping zones (📖 p. 205). A monitor zone is also available in the VT zone whereby detection occurs but no therapies are programmed. This can be used as a diagnostic tool to detect slower VTs. Before programming a device the answers to some important questions that will affect programming are required.

### Is the device for primary or secondary prevention?

Devices implanted for primary prevention will have to be programmed without any details of clinical arrhythmia.

### What clinical arrhythmias have been documented?

The most important question is what rate is the slowest ventricular arrhythmia as this will determine the VT zone. The VT zone is usually programmed to a cycle length (CL) 40–50ms longer than the slowest VT.

### How well is the VT tolerated?

With poorly tolerated VT (e.g. syncope, severe haemodynamic compromise), prompt treatment is required and a rapid progression to shock therapy is advisable. It is reasonable even with compromising fast VT to have one or two bursts of ATP as 70% of fast VT will respond.

### Is there a large amount of non-sustained VT?

Therapies for non-sustained VT are unnecessary as, by definition, the arrhythmia self-terminates. To avoid unnecessary therapies, detection time or number of intervals needed for detection may be increased (e.g. from nominal 12/16 intervals to 18/24).

### What are the results from EPS?

EPS may provoke VT that is clinically significant: note how haemodynamically tolerated it is (remembering the patient is supine) and its response to ATP.

## Programming for specific conditions

### Hypertrophic cardiomyopathy

These tend to be younger patients who are classified as high-risk based on LV wall thickness, syncope, non-sustained VT on Holter monitoring, family history, and poor blood pressure response to exercise. They are at risk of VT and also AF and so an atrial lead helps in terms of reducing risk of inappropriate therapies. SVT discriminators should be programmed 'on'. Dual chamber pacing may be used in cases of LVOT obstruction to improve haemodynamics, although this pacing indication remains controversial. Zones for VT and VF should be programmed, bearing in mind young patient may achieve fast ventricular rates with exercise and AF (despite beta blocker use).

### Brugada syndrome

Patients with Brugada syndrome are at risk of VF and/or polymorphic VT. These arrhythmias require shock therapy as they will not terminate with ATP. Slow detection rates are not usually required. An ICD may be implanted as a primary or secondary implant. There is also an association with SCN5A mutations and AF, so SVT discriminators should be programmed 'on'.

### Long QT syndrome

Patients with long QT syndrome are at risk of polymorphic VT, which may degenerate into VF. Often these are younger patients, who have had episodes of syncope or survived a cardiac arrest. Although devices may be programmed as a single VF zone, some studies have demonstrated polymorphic VT falling into a VT zone (< 208bpm or cycle length 288ms). Atrial pacing may be necessary to prevent pause-dependent arrhythmias so dual chamber devices are often recommended. Most patients will be on beta blockers; however their young age means fast ventricular rates may occur with exercise or other causes of sinus tachycardia.

## VF zone

- Every device has to have a VF zone with shocks. Detection rate is usually set at 200–240bpm (CL 300–250ms), depending upon other VT zones.
- Set as either time (e.g. 2s) or number of intervals (e.g. 12 of 16).
- SVT discriminators cannot be applied in this zone.
- The only therapy in this zone is shocks. Some operators start with a shock at DFT + 10J and then maximum output shocks; others advocate maximum output shocks from the onset. The advantage of a lower energy shock is a shorter charge-time. However, in modern devices charging to maximum output is rapid. The advantage of a maximum output shock is a higher probability of success. *All shocks are equally uncomfortable, regardless of the energy delivered.*

## Fast VT zone

- Detection rate is usually set 170–200bpm up to the VF zone.
- Set as either time (e.g. 5s) or number of intervals (e.g. 16).
- Therapies usually involve 1–2 bursts of ATP at 81–88% of the VT cycle length.
- After ATP, programmed to deliver shocks similarly to the VF zone.

## VT zone

- Detection rate is usually 150–170bpm up to the FVT zone.
- Set as either time (e.g. 10s) or number of intervals (e.g. 16).
- Therapies usually involve 4–8 bursts of ATP (some devices allow a mixture of burst and ramp).
- After ATP, programmed to deliver shock similarly to VF zone.

## SVT discriminators

These should be programmed on up to a rate of approximately 200bpm (CL 300ms). Depending on the device this may be programmed independently from the detection zones or in association with these (e.g. SVT discriminator in VT and FVT zones and *not* in VF zone).

Most devices have an option that overrides SVT discriminators after a programmable time interval, forcing VT detection and therapy even if the discriminators indicate SVT (Sustained rate duration, High Rate Timeout, Maximum Time to Diagnosis). These are usually programmed 'off' to avoid inappropriate therapies for SVTs.

### Example 1

- 78-year-old male: IHD, LVEF 20%, QRS duration 160ms, NYHA class I.
- Primary prevention; dual chamber ICD (MADIT II).

*Programming*
- DDI 40bpm. (No bradycardia pacing required and RV pacing may be detrimental to LV function.)
- VF 240bpm: maximum output shocks.
- FVT 188–240bpm (via VF criteria if available): 1–2 × ATP; then maximum output shocks.
- VT 167–188bpm: 6 × ATP; then maximum output shocks. (VT is frequently the initial arrhythmia in stable IHD.)

### Example 2

- 28-year-old male: LVEF 50%, Brugada syndrome, survived VF arrest.
- Secondary prevention: single chamber ICD.

*Programming*
- VVI/DDI 40bpm. (No bradycardia pacing required.)
- VF 222bpm: maximum output shocks.
- FVT 188bpm. 2 × ATP; then maximum output shocks. (Young patient may get sinus tachycardias up to 180+ bpm.)

### Example 3

- 76-year-old male: IHD, EF 25%, syncopal VT rate 155bpm.
- Secondary prevention: dual chamber ICD.

*Programming*
- DDI 40bpm.
- VF 240bpm: maximum output shocks.
- FVT 188–240bpm (via VF criteria if available). 1–2 × ATP; then maximum output shocks.
- VT 144–188: 6 × ATP; then maximum output shocks.

# Bradycardia pacing

In view of evidence, including the DAVID trial, demonstrating the detrimental effects of RV apical pacing in the ICD population, avoidance of RV pacing is recommended unless there is a standard indication for bradycardia pacing, e.g. complete heart block. One group of ICD patients in whom pacing may be therapeutic is patients with long QT syndrome in whom arrhythmias may be bradycardia- or pause-dependent. Atrial pacing may therefore help prevent arrhythmias and subsequent ICD therapies.

Most patients can therefore be set with only backup settings:
• VVI 40bpm;
• DDI 40bpm.

If there is a standard indication for programming this will be as explained previously (📖 p. 95). If the device is a CRT-D then programming will be to maintain biventricular pacing (📖 p. 306). If unsure consider using an ICD with AV search hysteresis or managed ventricular pacing.

# Post-shock pacing

In order to prevent long periods of asystole or bradycardia following shock therapy, post-shock pacing is used. Depending on the device this may have to be in the same mode as the bradycardia setting (e.g. DDD for both) or may be separate (e.g. AAIR for bradycardia pacing and DDD for post-shock pacing). The following parameters can be programmed.
• A programmable delay following shock therapy before pacing starts (usually 1–2s).
• Post-shock pacing will then continue for a programmed period before reverting to the bradycardia programmed rate and mode (usually 1min).
• Programmed to VVI or DDD (60–80bpm).

# Troubleshooting ICDs

# Assessing an ICD therapy

ICDs may deliver therapies appropriately (for genuine VT or VF) or inappropriately (for supraventricular arrhythmias or oversensing of intrinsic or external events). Therapies may also be withheld inappropriately, either through failure to detect (undersensing) or misclassification of ventricular arrhythmias as supraventricular arrhythmias. See Table 12.1 for characteristics of different arrhythmias.

Full interpretation of the event requires examination of stored EGMs and annotated markers. Ideally, the onset of the detected event and the effect(s) of therapies should be documented by the device.

## Response to therapy

Device therapies may result in one of the following.

### Appropriately delivered therapies
- Successful conversion of a ventricular tachyarrhythmia back to the patient's normal rhythm.
- Unsuccessful conversion of a ventricular tachyarrhythmia with continuation of the same tachycardia.
- Conversion of a ventricular arrhythmia into a different ventricular tachyarrhythmia.

### Inappropriately delivered therapies
- No effect on underlying sinus rhythm.
- Termination of a supraventricular arrhythmia.
- Pro-arrhythmia—initiation of a ventricular tachyarrhythmia.
- Pro-arrhythmia—initiation of a new supraventricular arrhythmia.

## Causes of inappropriate therapies

In response to a tachycardia:
- sinus tachycardia;
- atrial fibrillation/flutter;
- supraventricular tachycardia;
- non-sustained ventricular tachycardia.

During a rhythm with a normal ventricular rate:
- T-wave oversensing;
- double counting of ventricular depolarization;
- P-wave oversensing;
- external electromagnetic signals;
- lead failure or fracture.

**Table 12.1** Characteristics of different arrhythm as

| Rhythm | Onset | Stability | EGM morphology | A:V ratio | Effect of ATP | Effect of Shock |
|--------|-------|-----------|----------------|-----------|---------------|------------------|
| Sinus tachycardia | Gradual | Stable with subtle variations | Same as sinus rhythm | 1:1 | No effect* | No effect; may accelerate |
| Atrial flutter | Sudden; A before V | Stable† | Same as sinus rhythm‡ | A > V² | No effect* | May cardiovert to SR |
| Atrial fibrillation | Sudden: A before V | Irregular | Same as sinus rhythm‡ | A >> V | No effect* | May cardiovert to SR |
| Atrial tachycardia | Sudden: A before V | Stable‡ A–A variations precede V–V variations | Same as sinus rhythm‡ | A > V§ | No effect* | May cardiovert to SR |
| 'Junctional' SVT | Sudden | Stable | Same as sinus rhythm‡ | 1:1 | May terminate tachy | May cardiovert to SR |
| Monomorphic ventricular tachycardia | Sudden: V before A | Stable: subtle variations at onset | Different | V > A¶ | Often terminates tachy* | Usually cardioverts to SR |

* May be pro-arrhythmic † Unless variable AV block. ‡ Unless rate-related bundle branch block. § Unless 1:1 conduction to ventricle. ¶ Unless 1:1 VA conduction or coexisting atrial fibrillation/flutter

# Inappropriate therapies in response to tachycardia: introduction and sinus tachycardia

## Key information required

To assess appropriateness of therapy for a tachycardia gather the following information:

- EGM morphology before and after the therapy and during 'normal' rhythm (sensing EGM and shock coil EGM);
- response to therapy, including ventricular and atrial rates before and after the therapy;
- gradual or sudden onset;
- atrial and ventricular association (dual chamber devices only);
- stability.

## Sinus tachycardia

### Diagnosis

- Most commonly seen in young, physically active patients.
- Usually has a gradual onset and acceleration of heart rate.
- The sensing and shock EGMs should look identical to those during normal sinus rhythm (Fig. 12.1(a), (b)).
- There is a 1:1 relationship between atrium and ventricle in dual chamber devices. The PR interval is usually stable. There may be slight beat-to-beat fluctuations in cycle length. Note: ventricular premature beats during sinus tachycardia will result in V > A and the shorter cycle length may move detection into a higher zone.
- ATP usually has no effect on the subsequent tachycardia cycle length and may even be pro-arrhythmic. Shocks may cause sinus tachycardia to accelerate further, stay the same, or slow down.
- The cycle length in the atrial channel does not change during ATP (unless there is extremely good retrograde AV node conduction).

### Treatment

- Make sure SVT discriminators are on (especially onset, morphology, AV association, etc.).
- Avoid slow VT zones with detection rates close to physiological sinus tachycardia rates.
- Prescribe beta blockers to blunt the heart rate response.
- Assess effectiveness with exercise testing (therapies should be turned off).

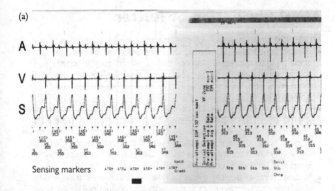

**Fig. 12.1(a)** Onset of sinus tachycardia. EGMs from A, atrial channel; V, ventricular channel; S, shock coil. The EGMs initially showing sinus tachycardia at 358ms (167bpm) with V sensing (VS in marker channel). These are recordings from a young patient with a dual chamber ECG who is exercising. There is sinus tachycardia (a gradual steady acceleration, the atrial rate = ventricular rate, and morphology is identical to sinus rhythm). As the rate increases above 170bpm (352ms) the tachycardia enters the VT detection zone (VT in marker channel). SVT discriminators are applied and therapies are withheld. However the sinus tachycardia accelerates further and, when the rate exceeds 190bpm (315ms), the tachycardia enters the VF zone (VF in the marker channel). SVT discriminators are not applied in the VF zone and charging begins.

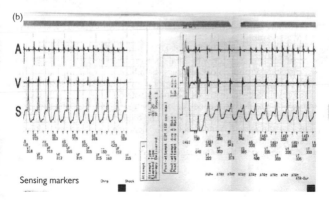

**Fig. 12.1(b)** Shock therapy for sinus tachycardia. Continuation from Fig. 12.1(a). A 41J shock is delivered. Sinus tachycardia continues, although at a slightly slower rate as the patient stops exercising. The rate falls within the VT zone and SVT discriminators withhold further therapies as the heart rate gradually slows.

# Atrial fibrillation or flutter

## Diagnosis

- A rapid ventricular rate during *atrial fibrillation* will be irregular (poor stability) with significant beat-to-beat variations in cycle length. Unfortunately, the faster the ventricular rate, the less dramatic the irregularity and, if it exceeds 170bpm, it may not fail the stability criteria (Fig. 12.2).
- *Typical atrial flutter* is usually regular with 2:1 conduction that is never greater than 150–160bpm (400ms CL). Atrial flutter may have 1:1 conduction, either in young patients with high sympathetic tone or in atypical flutters with slower atrial rates. If there is variable AV block the ventricular rate may be irregular. Onset is usually sudden with a short P–P interval preceding a short R–R interval.
- In dual chamber devices the atrial rate exceeds the ventricular rate (unless in the rare event of flutter with 1:1 conduction). In AF the atrial cycle lengths may be incredibly short (< 150ms). Beware of undersensing of atrial EGM during AF giving falsely slow rate.
- EGM morphology should be identical to that during normal rhythm unless there is new, rate-dependent bundle branch block. In patients with chronic AF, analysis of the atrial channel as part of the SVT discriminator is unhelpful (it will always show a very rapid atrial rate) and single chamber algorithms are used.
- ATP therapies usually have no effect on the rhythm or atrial rate, or may even be pro-arrhythmic. Shock therapies, however, may cardiovert flutter or fibrillation back into sinus rhythm.

## Treatment

- Make sure SVT discriminators are on (especially morphology, stability, AV association).
- Check that atrial sensitivity is adequate to detect the small amplitude atrial EGMs that occur with atrial fibrillation/flutter.
- Prescribe AV nodal blocking drugs (beta blockers, calcium channel blockers, digoxin) to slow the ventricular rate and/or anti-arrhythmics to prevent attacks (e.g. amiodarone or sotalol).
- Typical atrial flutter may be successfully treated with radiofrequency ablation. AF may be treated by ablating the AV node to create heart block—the patient is then pacemaker-dependent and the ventricular rate is controlled by the ICD.
- Consider appropriate anticoagulation strategies.

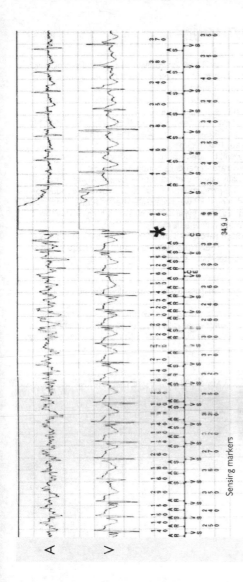

**Fig. 12.2** Inappropriate shock for atrial fibrillation. EGMs from A: atrial channel; V: ventricular channel. A very rapid, irregular cycle length (100–260ms) is seen in the atrial channel. The ventricular cycle length is fast enough to fall in the VT detection zone and, although irregular (240–360ms) at times, is stable enough to satisfy VT detection criteria. Also, at this rapid rate the ventricular electrogram morphology is variable and different from the sinus rhythm morphology (see after the shock). A 34.9J shock is delivered (*) that cardioverts the atrial fibrillation, restoring sinus tachycardia at a rate slower than the VT zone.

# Atrial tachycardia

### Diagnosis

- Less common than atrial flutter or fibrillation, atrial tachycardia has a sudden onset (although it may accelerate further). At onset, a short P–P interval precedes a short R–R interval.
- It is generally regular, although small variations in the P–P interval may precede variations in the R–R interval.
- There is often a 1:1 relationship. However there may be periods of AV Wenckebach or 2:1 block during which the ventricular rate falls below the atrial rate (Fig. 12.3(a)).
- EGM morphology will be identical to that during normal rhythm unless there is new rate-dependent bundle branch block.
- ATP therapies usually have no effect on the overall rhythm or atrial rate, or may even be pro-arrhythmic. Rarely, retrograde conduction up the AV node during ATP will accelerate the atrial rate and terminate tachycardia. If tachycardia terminates during ATP without a change in the atrial cycle length the diagnosis is VT.
- Shock therapies often cardiovert atrial tachycardia back into sinus rhythm (Fig. 12.3(b)). There may be a very rapid re-initiation of atrial tachycardia immediately post-shock.

### Treatment

- Make sure SVT discriminators are on (especially morphology and AV association).
- Prevent atrial tachycardia with anti-arrhythmic drugs (amiodarone, sotalol) or slow the ventricular rate (beta blockers, verapamil).
- Some atrial tachycardias may be treated with radiofrequency ablation.

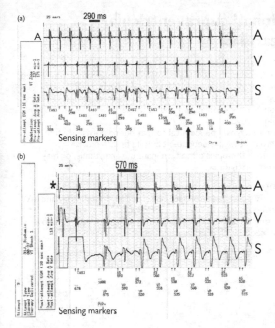

**Fig. 12.3** Atrial tachycardia. EGMs from A, Atrial channel; V, ventricular channel; S, shock coil. (a) There is a regular atrial tachycardia, CL 290ms (207/bpm) with variable conduction to the ventricle with a Wenckebach-type pattern resulting in an irregular ventricular rate. R–R intervals fall within the VT zone (VT in the marker channel) and VF zone (VF in the marker channel, arrow). Although V > A and the ventricular rate is not stable, the morphology is very variable (rate-dependent aberrancy) and entering the VF zone prohibits the use of SVT discriminators.
(b) Shock for atrial tachycardia. Continuation from Fig. 12.3(a): shock therapy converts the atrial tachycardia back to sinus rhythm (570ms, 105bpm) with atrial sensing and ventricular pacing and the episode finishes.

# 'Junctional' supraventricular tachycardias

### Diagnosis

- It is very unusual to see junctional SVTs (accessory pathway-mediated tachycardias or AV nodal re-entrant tachycardia) in the ICD population. They are characterized by sudden onset with a 1:1 relationship between atrium and ventricle.
- The rhythm is regular.
- EGM morphology will be identical to that during normal rhythm unless there is new rate-dependent bundle branch block.
- ATP and shock therapies often terminate the arrhythmia, or may rarely be pro-arrhythmic.

### Treatment

- Make sure SVT discriminators are on (especially morphology and AV association).
- Drug treatment (beta blockers, calcium channel blockers) has now been superseded with curative radiofrequency ablation.

**Reasons that SVT discriminators may fail to identify SVTs/AF**

- Very rapidly conducted AF is relatively stable (stability satisfies VT criteria).
- Postventricular atrial blanking (to eliminate far-field R-wave sensing) may blank too many atrial EGMs making A < V (atrial undersensing).
- Undersensing of small atrial EGMs during AF.
- Rate-dependent bundle branch block may change EGM morphology.
- Ventricular rate fast enough to fall into VF zone, where SVT discriminators are not applied.
- Ventricular ectopics make V > A and also affect morphology criteria.

**General approaches to overcome inappropriate therapies for SVT**

- Adjust SVT discriminators (turn more on, change settings). Remember that increasing the sensitivity for SVTs decreases the specificity and raises the chances of withholding appropriate therapies for VT. SVT discriminators will not be applied in the VF zone, however.
- Programme in more VT zones and more ATP. Make VF zone faster (e.g. 250bpm rather than 188bpm).
- Relearn a new sinus rhythm EGM morphology template.
- In patients with sinus rhythm and single chamber ICDs, upgrade to a dual chamber device to add an extra discriminator.
- Anti-arrhythmic drugs or ablation to prevent SVTs and control ventricular response.

# Non-sustained ventricular tachycardia (NSVT) and frequent ventricular ectopy

## Diagnosis

Delivering therapies for NSVT is not due to inappropriate or incorrect discrimination, but rather a failure to recognize that the arrhythmia self-terminates (Fig. 12.4). If NSVT starts, stops, and restarts spontaneously, it is likely to continue doing so after ATP or shocks. Short charge times now mean that confirmation and redetection happen relatively quickly. Confirmation algorithms will deliver an initial shock if a few sensed intervals immediately after charging fall within the detection zone. If NSVT has terminated during charging, sinus tachycardia, ventricular ectopics, or a further episode of NSVT may allow confirmation and cause the shock to be delivered, particularly if there in a slow VT zone. Subsequent shocks will be committed (no confirmation after charging) and so delayed termination of VT or VF after a therapy may lead to inappropriate 2nd or 3rd therapies.

Ventricular ectopic beats, particularly during sinus tachycardia that enters a slow VT zone, may be enough to override SVT discriminators as they will make the V count greater than the A count and will have a different EGM morphology from sinus rhythm.

## Treatment

- Patients with known NSVT or VF (particularly common in dilated cardiomyopathy and long-QT patients) should have longer detection time criteria programmed in to give the arrhythmia time to terminate before detection criteria are satisfied (e.g. 18 out of 24 intervals rather than the nominal 12 out of 16 intervals).
- Increasing redetection times or criteria may prevent inappropriate 2nd or 3rd therapies that occur due to delayed termination.
- Excessive delays, however, make the occurrence of syncope more likely.
- Also, longer times to defibrillation result in higher DFTs and lower the chance of success.

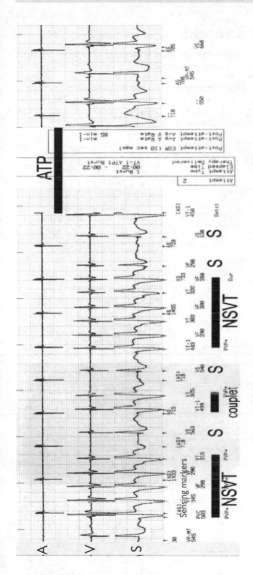

**Fig. 12.4** Inappropriate therapy for non-sustained VT (NSVT). EGMs from A, Atrial channel; V, ventricular channel; S, shock coil. There is a 5 beat run of NSVT, a sinus beat (S), a ventricular couplet, a sinus beat, a 6 beat run of NSVT, two sinus beats, and ATP is finally triggered by a premature ventricular beat.

# Committed shocks

In some devices, confirmation of the rhythm after charging only takes place for the first shock therapy. Once the first shock has been delivered, if the device detects ongoing tachycardia, further therapies are committed, i.e. once charging is completed there is no confirmation and therefore the therapy is delivered even if the tachycardia stopped during charging (as may happen with delayed conversion, when VT or VF terminates a few seconds after the shock is delivered; Fig. 12.5(a), (b)).

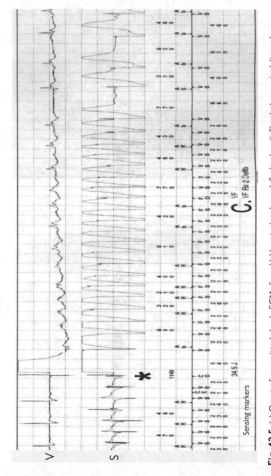

**Fig. 12.5** (a) Onset of committed shock. EGMs from V, Ventricular channel; S, shock coil. Shock therapy is delivered appropriately for ventricular tachycardia (*). This accelerates the tachycardia for 21 beat run with a different morphology before delayed termination and sinus rhythm. Unfortunately, redetection occurs (C), before the delayed termination and charging begins.

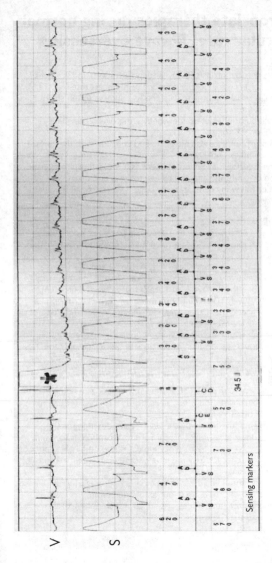

**Fig. 12.5** (b) Committed shock. Continuation of Fig. 12.5(a). As the second shock is committed, there is no confirmation of the rhythm and a 34.5J shock is delivered (*) despite the rhythm being sinus rhythm. This results in a transient sinus tachycardia with distorted EGM morphology that gradually slows and is below the VT detection rate, so there is no redetection.

# Inappropriate therapies during normal ventricular rate: T-wave oversensing

## Diagnosis

- The device detects intrinsic R waves (depolarization) and T waves (repolarization) causing double counting of the heart rate (Fig. 12.6).
- R–R intervals usually alternate, with the R–T interval often shorter than the T–R interval.
- The interval durations determine whether the oversensing falls into the VF or VT zones.
- The EGM morphologies also alternate and coincide with the surface ECG QRS complex and T wave.
- T-wave oversensing may be intermittent as T-wave morphology and size can be dynamic and affected by electrolytes and drugs.
- It may occur following comparatively large R waves, small R waves, or post-pacing.

## Treatment

- As with any oversensing problem, decreasing a device's sensitivity (increasing the minimum R-wave value for detection) runs the risk of undersensing true VT or VF.
- If the intrinsic R wave is very large (e.g. > 10mV) and the T-wave amplitude is relatively small (e.g. 1.0mV), decreasing the sensitivity to just greater than the T wave (e.g. 1.2mV) may solve the problem.
- Alternatively, it may be possible to programme the ventricular channel autogain or extend the maximum and minimum values and slope of the decay to avoid T-wave sensing (📖 p. 202).
- If T-wave oversensing occurs *only after pacing* it may affect bradycardia pacing but should not result in inappropriate therapies (only the T waves are ventricular sensed events). It should be possible to extend the post-pacing ventricular blanking period without compromising arrhythmia detection.
- If T-wave oversensing occurs after sensed R waves, extending the ventricular blanking period is not advisable as it is likely to lead to undersensing of VT or VF.
- Alternate events (the R waves) should be a good match for the morphology discriminator algorithm. Turning morphology 'on' will classify the rhythm as an SVT (in St Jude ICDs, the nominal number of morphology matches for SVT must be decreased from 5 to 4 to reject T-wave oversensing).
- A VF induction should be performed to check sensing of VF and make sure there is not excessive drop-out and undersensing.
- If the R- and T-wave amplitudes are similar, repositioning of the ventricular lead may be required.

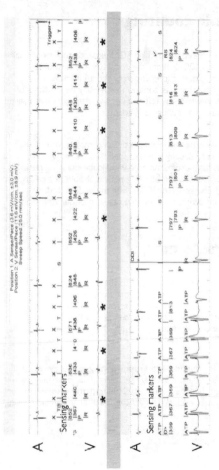

**Fig. 12.6** T-wave oversensing. ECMs from A, Atrial channel; V, ventricular channel. During sinus rhythm there is T-wave oversensing (*) and double counting of the ventricular rate. The T waves are small (and not all are sensed) but so are the R waves, making it more difficult to discriminate between the two with R-wave sensitivity programming. The sensed R–R interval shows the typical alternating cycle length of R–T (approximately 438ms) and T–R (approximately 406ms). Neither the small, intrinsic R wave nor the T wave match the morphology of the sinus rhythm template EGM (X). ATP is delivered; then sinus rhythm continues. However the PR interval now prolongs, the R wave amplitude is much greater, the morphology matches, and the T waves are no longer sensed.

## Oversensing

Oversensing refers to the presence of additional events other than the initial depolarization detected in the sensing electrodes of the ventricular channel. When the intervals between registered events are short enough to fall into arrhythmia detection windows, therapies may be initiated. In pacing-dependent patients, oversensing may also lead to inappropriate inhibition of ventricular pacing (□ p. 138).

# R-wave double counting

### Diagnosis
- If the duration of the sensed ventricular EGM exceeds the ventricular blanking period (usually 120–140ms), the local R wave is double counted. There are alternating long and very short intervals.
- This type of double counting was common with early generations of biventricular devices in which the left and right ventricular leads shared a common ventricular port through a Y-adapter.

### Treatment
- Altering the sensitivity is not usually effective and may lead to undersensing. Treatment usually requires lead repositioning.
- Most devices do not have programmable ventricular blanking periods but, if this feature is possible, the blanking period should not be greater than 140–150ms; otherwise VT or VF may be underdetected.
- Decreasing ventricular sensitivity may also result in underdetection of ventricular arrhythmias.

# P-wave oversensing

### Diagnosis
- If the ventricular lead is positioned close to the tricuspid valve annulus and it has an integrated bipole (the proximal pole is the distal RV shocking coil), there may be P-wave oversensing. This is more likely to happen in children or patients with a septal lead position.
- There is double counting in sinus rhythm and there may be dramatic oversensing with AF or atrial flutter.

### Treatment
- As for R-wave double counting. Lead repositioning is usually required.
- An alternative is to force atrial pacing (e.g. using atrial overdrive pacing algorithms), provided that the shorter cycle length and cross-chamber ventricular blanking after each atrial event stop far-field P-wave sensing.

# External interference

## Diagnosis

- External interference (noise) usually appears as very high frequency signals with no isoelectric baseline. If there is a shocking coil EGM available it is usually of greater amplitude than the sensing EGM from the distal, closely spaced electrodes.
- Another example of high frequency external signals is myopotentials, usually from the diaphragm, and often occurring after long diastolic periods or ventricular paced events, when amplifier gain is maximal. Myopotentials are therefore most likely to occur with integrated bipolar leads positioned in the RV apex in devices with an automatic gain function.

## Treatment

- Avoid the external interference. If the patient is employed, a site visit to the workplace may be required to identify the source of electromagnetic interference.
- If there is myopotential oversensing, lead repositioning may be required.

# Lead damage/loose connection

## Diagnosis

- A fractured lead or loose connector or set screw may cause intermittent artefact (Fig. 12.7(a)) that can sometimes be reproduced by movement or generator manipulation.
- The pacing impedance may be abnormal (intermittent or continuous).
- The high frequency artefact can be interpreted as VF and result in inappropriate therapies.

## Treatment

- Usually lead extraction and replacement.
- If the shock coils function correctly an additional pace-sense lead may be added without removing the fractured ICD lead.

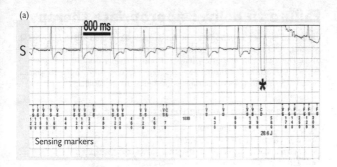

(a)

**800 ms**

S

Sensing markers

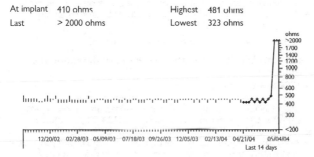

(b)                     Lead performance trends report

**Ventricular pacing impedance**

| | | | |
|---|---|---|---|
| At implant | 410 ohms | Highest | 481 ohms |
| Last | > 2000 ohms | Lowest | 323 ohms |

ohms
>2000
1700
1400
1200
1000
800
600
500
400
300
<200

12/20/02  02/28/03  05/09/03  07/18/03  09/26/03  12/05/03  02/13/04  04/21/04  05/04/04

Last 14 days

**Fig. 12.7** (a) Lead damage. S, Shock coil. It can be clearly seen that the ventricular rate is 75bpm (800ms) yet there are many rapid ventricular sensed events at extremely short R–R intervals (e.g. 120ms) that cause the device to deliver a shock for VF (*). (b) Lead impedance record for patient in (a). There is a sudden dramatic increase in impedance to > 2000 ohms which coincides with the lead fracture and onset of inappropriate shocks.

# Failure to deliver appropriate therapy

Failure to deliver appropriate therapies may have fatal consequences. In general, ICD design and algorithms err on the side of caution and are more likely to deliver therapy inappropriately than withhold therapy inappropriately. Some algorithms (e.g. sustained rate duration) are specifically aimed at preventing inappropriate withholding of therapies.

## Reasons why appropriate therapies not delivered

- Therapies are switched off.
- Tachycardia is in a monitor zone.
- Tachycardia is slower than minimum detection rate.
- Tachycardia is incorrectly identified as SVT.
- Undersensing (tachycardia is not detected).
- Tachycardia undetected through bradycardia pacing blanking periods.

## Inactivation of the ICD

### Diagnosis

- ICD therapies may be deliberately turned off (monitor-only) when patients undergo surgery in order to avoid inappropriate shocks during diathermy. Therapies must be programmed back on after procedure.
- A strong magnet positioned over the ICD generator temporarily suspends therapies (📖 p. 354).

*Treatment* Make sure therapies are programmed on!

## Tachycardia is slower than the minimum detection rate

### Diagnosis

- ICDs only detect arrhythmias within the programmed detection zones. Slow VT, undetected by the device, usually comes to light through patient symptoms (palpitations, breathlessness, dizziness, or chest pains) or ECG Holter monitors. Sustained, slow VT may cause severe heart failure symptoms in patients with poor LV function.
- Anti-arrhythmic drugs, particularly amiodarone and class 1 drugs, slow ventricular rates, which may take them below VT detection.
- A VT cycle length that fluctuates, crossing up into and down out of the slow VT zone, will be interpreted as non-sustained VT.
- Rarely, device therapies may convert a rapid VT into a slow VT that is below the detection zone (Fig. 12.8).
- Have a high index of suspicion for the presence of slow VT in patients with severe heart failure on anti-arrhythmic drugs.

### Treatment

- Programme a slow VT zone. The slow VT detection cycle length intervals should be at least 40–50ms longer than the slowest documented or induced VT.

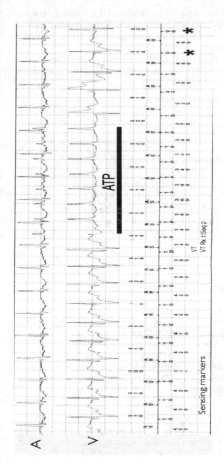

**Fig. 12.8** Tachycardia drops below detection rate. EGMs from A, Atrial channel; V, ventricular channel. A slow VT (cycle length 390–450ms, 133–154bpm; TS in marker channel) with a sinus rhythm cycle length of 510ms (117bpm) is detected within the slow VT zone of 460ms (130bpm). ATP is delivered (black line), which slows the VT to 490ms cycle length (122bpm, *) while the sinus rate continues at 117bpm. This is below the detection rate and is no longer classified as VT by the device (VS in marker channel).

- If there is concern at very slow VT rates about inappropriate detection of sinus tachycardia, SVTs, or AF, make sure SVT discriminators are programmed on. It is usually possible to programme ATP only (no shocks) in slow VT zones.
- If slow VT cannot be suppressed with drug therapy and continues to be a problem. then radiofrequency ablation of the VT circuit should be considered.

### Tachycardia in the monitor zone

*Diagnosis* Slow VT zones may be programmed to 'monitor-only' and used to detect the presence of slow VT, but not deliver any therapies.

*Treatment* Programme ATP, or ATP and shocks, into the slow VT zone.

### Inappropriate classification of VT as SVT

#### Diagnosis

- Therapies may be delayed or withheld if SVT discriminator criteria inappropriately classify VT as SVT. Ventricular tachycardia may begin with irregular R–R intervals before settling into a regular rhythm. Polymorphic VT and VF will be irregular, although they have much shorter cycle lengths (usually in the VF zone, where SVT discriminators are not applied).
- Stability algorithms at nominal setting misclassify VT as AF in < 0.5% of cases. Morphology algorithms misclassify VT as SVT in 1–5% of cases when used alone. Onset criteria may also misclassify VT as SVT in 1–2% of cases if the VT gradually accelerates across zones. These algorithms are much more accurate when combined with dual chamber sensing, comparing the atrial to the ventricular rate.
- If the atrial lead displaces into the ventricle, or there is a large far-field R wave in the atrial channel, ventricular events will be sensed in the atrial and ventricular channels causing A = V or A > V.
- A 1:1 AV relationship will withhold treatment if it is the only SVT discriminator programmed on. If there is 1:1 retrograde conduction from ventricle to atrium there will be a 1:1 relationship. This is more likely to occur with slower VTs.

#### Treatment

- If SVT discriminators are required, programme them such that more than one (or all) have to be satisfied for SVT to be diagnosed and therapy withheld, rather than just one. Overall, it is probably better to receive an inappropriate shock for SVT than have therapies withheld during VT.
- Duration-based safety features (sustained rate duration (SRD), high rate timeout, maximum time to diagnosis (MTD)) are available that override SVT classification if the ventricular rate remains in the detection zone for longer than a programmed period of time (e.g. 2min). These features anticipate that sinus tachycardia, AF, or other SVTs will only reach the detection rate for transient, short periods before the ventricular rate slows, whereas VT will continue to remain within the detection zone. At the end of the programmed time, therapy is delivered. Programming these functions 'on' increases the risk of inappropriate therapies.

# Undersensing

## Diagnosis

Undersensing occurs when the amplitude of ventricular EGM is below that required to register a sensed event. It may occur in the following situations.

- *Complete sensing failure.* R wave during sinus rhythm and tachycardias is too small to be detected. Not only will there be failure to detect tachycardia, but there will also be inappropriate bradycardia pacing.
- *Sensing failure during tachycardia.* The R waves during VF (or, less frequently, VT) are too small to be detected, whereas R waves during sinus rhythm are large enough to be detected. VF may have rapid variations in R-wave amplitude. If there are consecutive EGMs that are too small to be detected (dropout), the cycle length measurements may fall below the tachycardia detection zone and the device could interpret this as tachycardia termination and normal ventricular activation (Fig. 12.9).
- *Post-shock undersensing.* More common with integrated bipolar leads.
- *Programming failure.* Decreasing the ventricular sensitivity (e.g. to avoid T-wave oversensing) increases the chance of undersensing small amplitude ventricular EGMs.
- *Blanking of ventricular events during high rate bradycardia pacing.* During high-rate, atrial, or dual-chamber pacing, sensing may be restricted to short periods of the cardiac cycle because of the combined effects of ventricular blanking after ventricular pacing and cross-chamber ventricular blanking after atrial pacing, which is needed to avoid cross-talk. Algorithms such as rate-smoothing (📖 p. 97) may promote high-rate pacing.

## Treatment

- It is rare to completely undersense VF if the intrinsic R-wave amplitude during sinus rhythm is > 5mV. Ventricular sensitivity should be set to the least sensitive setting (usually 0.3mV) and detection tested at the time of implant or whenever the sensing lead is changed.
- Programming functions such as autogain or dynamic adjustment of sensitivity may help, although rarely can cause undersensing (i.e. decreasing sensitivity after consecutive large amplitude R waves may result in undersensing of small amplitude R waves that occur immediately afterwards).
- Shorter blanking periods may need to be programmed.
- If there is failure to sense correctly during normal sinus rhythm, lead repositioning or addition of a new pace-sense lead is required.

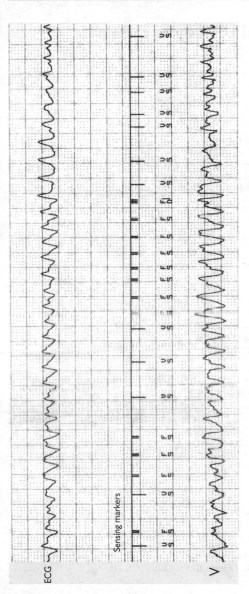

**Fig. 12.9** Undersensing of VF. The ECG tracing shows VF. The marker channel, however, demonstrates that there is undersensing, with some ventricular EGMs not detected by the device. When adjacent EGMs are sensed, the counters register VF (FS). When some are missed, the corresponding sensed R–R interval is below the VF detection rate and therefore they register as ventricular sensed events rather than tachycardia (VS).

# Failure of therapy to terminate tachycardia

ICDs may fail to terminate a detected arrhythmia for the following reasons:
- inappropriate classification of an SVT as VT;
- failure to defibrillate VT or VF;
- probabilistic failure;
- high defibrillation threshold due to ischaemia, electrolyte disturbance, drug effects;
- lead or device failure;
- failure of ATP to terminate VT;
- acceleration or change in morphology;
- ongoing VT of same morphology;
- immediate reinitiation of ventricular arrhythmia (failure to recognize termination).

## Shock failure

### Diagnosis
- Defibrillation is *probabilistic*, so single shocks occasionally fail to convert ventricular tachycardia or fibrillation back to sinus rhythm, even at maximum output. Failure may be an alteration in tachycardia (Fig. 12.10), or complete lack of effect. If there is an adequate safety margin, however, consecutive shocks should not fail.
- Patient-related factors that lead to an increase in the defibrillation threshold include significant ventricular dilatation, ischaemia and further infarction, electrolyte imbalances (especially $K^+$), and anti-arrhythmic drugs (e.g. amiodarone).
- Pleural or pericardial effusions will shunt current away from the heart.
- Prolonged arrhythmia episodes may lead to ischaemia and further increases in the DFT.
- Generator migration around the chest wall may change the shock vector, affecting thresholds.

### Treatment
- If the change in DFT is due to a reversible causes (drugs, electrolytes, etc.) this should be corrected.
- If there is a long delay in delivering shock therapy, reducing or avoiding ineffective ATP and appropriate detection programming are necessary.
- If there are no reversible causes, some devices (St Jude) allow programming of the shock waveform. It may be possible to change the shock vector by programming (St Jude) or by physically unplugging the SVC coil (p. 219).
- The ventricular lead may need to be repositioned (e.g. into the RV outflow tract) or a new coil added.
- Lead or other component failure will require surgical revision.
- After changing anti-arrhythmic drug prescriptions, or whenever there is cause for concern, further DFT testing should be performed to assess the safety margin (p. 230).

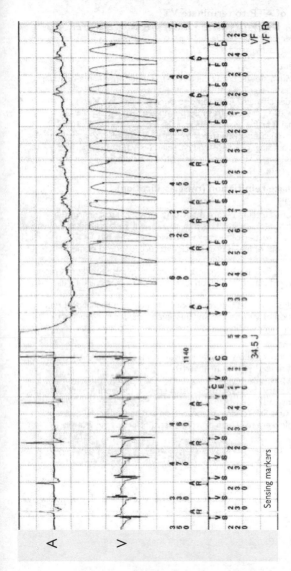

**Fig. 12.10** Shock fails to terminate VT. ECGs from A, Atrial channel; V, ventricular channel. Ventricular tachycardia with a 240ms cycle length has been detected. A 34.5J shock fails to restore sinus rhythm and tachycardia is seen to continue (with post-shock alteration of EGM morphology).

## Failure of ATP to terminate VT

*Diagnosis* If ATP fails to terminate correctly identified VT, tachycardia will either continue unaffected or may be altered to a faster or slower ventricular tachycardia (Fig. 12.11).

*Treatment*
- VTs with a slow CL may need ATP to be performed at a relatively faster rate (e.g. 70% of VT CL rather than 88%).
- Consider changing from ramp to burst pacing or vice versa.
- ATP with 12 or 15 pulses may be more effective than the nominal 6 or 8.
- If ATP repeatedly fails to terminate fast VT that is haemodynamically compromising, or consistently accelerates VT, or degenerates VT into VF, avoiding ATP and going straight to shock therapy is probably more appropriate.

## Immediate reinitiation (misclassification)

*Diagnosis*
- If VT or VF recurs before the ICD has had time to confirm the restoration of a normal rhythm, therapy will be classified as ineffective and the next tier of therapy will begin.
- The main problem is post-shock detection of non-sustained VT, which may lead to inappropriate delivery of an additional shock(s). This is more likely to occur in Medtronic devices with 'Smart-mode' (perceived failure of ATP on four occasions inhibits further use of ATP).
- Post-therapy sinus tachycardia or SVTs may lead to inappropriate detection of VT and ongoing therapies. Changes in cycle length, morphology stability, and VA association may point to this.

*Treatment*
- Some devices allow programming to decrease the time taken to detect sinus rhythm post-therapy.
- When possible, programming multiple tiers of ATP may avoid unnecessary shocks for non-sustained ATP (delivering painless ATP instead).
- Make sure SVT discriminators are on and applied to redetection.
- Beta blockers may help prevent post-shock sinus tachycardia.

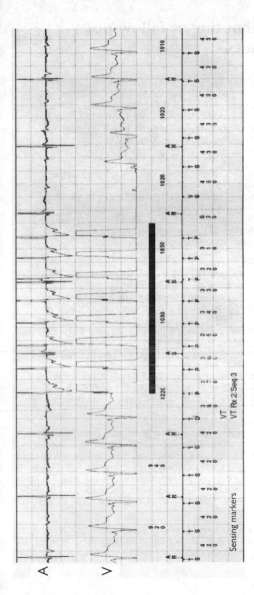

**Fig. 12.11** Failure of ATP to terminate ventricular tachycardia. ECGs from A, Atrial channel; V, ventricular channel. Ventricular tachycardia with a 420ms cycle length has been detected. An eight beat burst of ATP (black line) fails to restore sinus rhythm as the tachycardia continues at the same rate.

# Troubleshooting at follow-up: other issues

## Battery life

- ICD batteries have slightly different behaviour from pacemaker batteries (which tend to demonstrate a gradual, consistently slow decline in unloaded cell voltage). ICD batteries have capacitor charging characteristics that may also be measured. For the first 1/3 of their lifespan, battery voltage stays around 3.0V before dropping fairly rapidly to 2.6V. It then plateaus for 50–60% of its lifespan. As it reaches end-of life, the battery voltage drops further (although not by much) and capacitor charge times increase.
- Premature battery depletion is not uncommon. It may follow excessive capacitor charging or discharging, a high percentage of bradycardia pacing (especially if at high output), or lead insulation problems. Battery drain is also increased when multiple diagnostic features are in continual use. VT or VF storms with large numbers of shocks may also lead to battery depletion.
- Treatment is generator replacement.

## Lead problems

- Lead failure may manifest as failure to sense, inappropriate detection, failure to pace, or failure to deliver effective therapy.
- Occasionally it may manifest as asymptomatic artefact on stored intracardiac EGM or an abnormal impedance reading at routine follow-up ((📖 p. 134).
- ICD leads are more complex and thicker in diameter and are more prone to fracture and crush injuries.
- In dual chamber devices, atrial lead failure may result in failure of some SVT discriminators.
- Shock voltage impedance is normally 25–75 ohms. Painless testing of the shock impedance can check shock coil integrity.
- If lead damage is suspected, chest radiography is recommended to look for visible signs of fracture.
- Treatment is usually lead replacement.
- An alternative strategy for patients in whom lead extraction is deemed high risk is the addition of a single ventricular pace-sense lead. The new lead tip needs to be positioned away from the damaged ICD lead (e.g. an active fixation lead screwed into the RVOT) and plugged into the generator IS-1 ventricular pace-sense port. This option is only available if there is adequate venous access to insert a new lead and the integrity of the shock coils in the damaged lead can be confirmed.

**Audible alerts** Some devices have audible alerts (beeps) that notify the patient if there is a detected abnormality in lead impedance or battery life, long charge times, or more than three shocks in one episode.

# Cardiac resynchronization therapy (CRT)

# Background

Continuous pacing stimulation of the RV apex has been shown to be deleterious to myocardial function. For this reason, pacemaker therapy has previously been avoided in patients with heart failure. Recently this view has changed and pacing therapies for selected patients with heart failure have shown improvements in cardiac performance, symptoms, and, more recently, potential mortality benefit.

Left bundle branch block (LBBB) indicates electrical dyssynchrony and, in association with poor LV function, is an independent risk factor for morbidity and mortality. Increasing QRS width has been correlated with greater mortality. LBBB often correlates with mechanical dyssynchrony, i.e. non-physiological timing of LV and RV contraction, and thus interventricular delay. There may also be abnormal contraction of individual segments of the LV causing intraventricular delay. With significant impairment of LV function this can have a major impact on cardiac performance. It is not known whether the effects of dyssynchronous contraction cause disease progression or reflect the disease state.

Cardiac resynchronization therapy (CRT) aims to restore or improve ventricular contraction by stimulating both RV and LV (biventricular pacing) in symptomatic patients. Approximately one-third of patients with systolic dysfunction will have QRS durations greater than 120ms (usually LBBB; see Fig. 13.1). This results in delayed LV contraction through the septum after RV contraction often with a delayed lateral wall.

## Haemodynamic effects of ventricular dyssynchrony

- Mitral valve abnormalities:
  - delayed mitral valve opening;
  - distorted mitral valve annulus;
  - mitral regurgitation (including presystolic).
- Aortic valve abnormalities:
  - delayed aortic valve opening and closing.
- LV abnormalities:
  - abnormal septal motion;
  - reduced duration of LV filling;
  - decreased cardiac output (CO), ejection fraction (EF), mean arterial pressure (MAP);
  - increased end systolic volume.

Placement of a lead in the LV cavity would carry unacceptable risks of thromboembolism and may impair aortic valve function. Cardiac resynchronization is therefore achieved by stimulation of the LV via the cardiac veins. These are readily accessible via the coronary sinus and traverse the epicardial surface. The alternative is placing an electrode on the LV epicardium via a thoracotomy. This carries additional associated morbidity and mortality compared to a purely endocardial approach.

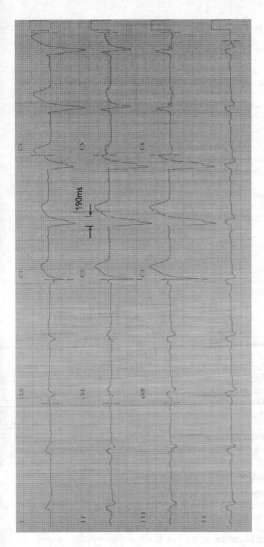

**Fig. 13.1** LBBB with a long QRS duration of 190ms and first degree heart block with PR interval of 280ms.

# Evidence base for CRT

The first studies of CRT were published in the mid-1990s and consisted of a number of acute and chronic observational studies. Initial studies utilized epicardial pacing leads followed by conventional endocardial pacing leads placed in the coronary venous system, and, finally, custom designed leads. Since this time a number of large multicentre randomized studies have examined the effects of CRT. A number of different end points have been assessed. Table 13.1 summarizes the outcomes of some of these studies.

### End points
- New York Heart Association (NYHA) classification.
- 6 minute walk test.
- $VO_2$ max.
- Quality of life.
- Hospitalization for heart failure.
- Ejection fraction.
- Mortality.

Early studies were positive in terms of morbidity but later studies have supported an improvement in mortality. The issues are complicated by the fact that CRT can exist as a pacing therapy alone (CRT-P) or in combination with an implantable cardioverter–defibrillator (CRT-D). It is important to recognize that CRT is not an alternative to medical therapy and should be considered as an adjunct to conventional medical therapy. This means that all patients should be thoroughly investigated for reversible causes.

### Positive effects of CRT
Mechanisms for the positive effects of CRT include:
- improved diastolic LV filling;
- increased EF, cardiac output (CO), dP/dT;
- reduced mitral regurgitation, left atrial pressure;
- reversed LV remodelling (not just a direct affect of pacing as the improved function and cardiac dimensions continue after CRT is turned off);
- improved neurohormonal balance, e.g. BNP;
- restoration of autonomic imbalance, e.g. heart rate variability.

### Key information from evidence base
- QRS complexes generally very wide (> 160ms).
- Most data applied to NYHA III & IV.
- Universal morbidity benefit demonstrated.
- Only studies to demonstrate mortality benefit (COMPANION and CARE-HF) had combined end points rather than mortality alone.

**Table 13.1** Summary of major studies of CRT

| Study | N | NYHA class | QRS (ms) | LVEF (%) | Key outcomes (= improvements in) |
|---|---|---|---|---|---|
| PATH-CHF[1] | 42 | III or IV | 175 ± 32 | 21 ± 7 | VO₂max, 6min walk test, NYHA, QOL |
| MUSTIC[2] | 47 | III or IV | 176 ± 19 | 23 ± 7 | VO₂max, 6min walk test, NYHA, QOL, hospitalization |
| MIRACLE3 | 453 | III or IV | 165 ± 20 | 22 ± 6 | VO₂max, 6min walk test, NYHA, QOL, exercise time, LVEF, hospitalization |
| MIRACLE ICD[4] | 555 | II–IV | 164 | 21 ± 7 | NYHA, QOL, exercise time |
| CONTAK-CD[5] | 490 | II–IV | 160 ± 27 | 22 ± 7 | VO₂max, 6min walk test, NYHA, QOL |
| COMPANION[6] | 1520 | III or IV | 160 | 21 | Combined end point of death & hospitalization |
| CARE HF[7] | 813 | III or IV | 160 | 25 | Combined end point of death & hospitalization, symptoms, QOL, MR, LVEF |

QOL, Quality of life; MR, mitral regurgitation.

1 Stellbrink C, et al.: PATH-CHF (PAcing THerapies in Congestive Heart Failure) investigators; CPI Guidant Congestive Heart Failure Research Group (2001). Impact of cardiac resynchronization therapy using hemodynamically optimized pacing on left ventricular remodeling in patients with congestive heart failure and ventricular conduction disturbances. J Am Coll Cardiol 38 (7), 1957–65. 2 Cazeau S, et al.: Multisite Stimulation in Cardiomyopathies (MUSTIC) study investigators (2001). Effects of multisite biventricular pacing in patients with heart failure and intraventricular conduction delay. N Engl J Med 344 (12), 873–80. 3 Abraham WT, et al.; MIRACLE Study Group. Multicenter InSync Randomized Clinical Evaluation (2002). Cardiac resynchronization in chronic heart failure. N Engl J Med 346 (24), 845–53. 4 Young JB, et al.: Multicenter InSync ICD Randomized Clinical Evaluation (MIRACLE ICD) trial investigators (2003). Combined cardiac resynchronization and implantable cardioversion defibrillation in advanced chronic heart failure: the MIRACLE ICD Trial. J Am Med Assoc 289 (20), 2685–94. 5 Higgins SL, et al. (2003). Cardiac resynchronization therapy for the treatment of heart failure in patients with intraventricular conduction delay and malignant ventricular tachyarrhythmias. J Am Coll Cardiol 42 (8), 1454–9. 6 Bristow MR, et al.: Comparison of Medical Therapy, Pacing, and Defibrillation in Heart Failure (COMPANION) investigators (2004). Cardiac-resynchronization therapy with or without an implantable defibrillator in advanced chronic heart failure. N Engl J Med 350 (21), 2140–50. 7 Cleland JG, et al.: Cardiac Resynchronization–Heart Failure (CARE-HF) study investigators (2005). The effect of cardiac resynchronization on morbidity and mortality in heart failure. N Engl J Med 352 (15), 1539–49.

## Indications for CRT

On the basis of the evidence patients with all of the following fundamental findings should be considered for CRT:
- patients on stable optimal medical management;
- symptomatic patients in NYHA III or IV;
- LVEF ≤ 35%;
- LV end-diastolic diameter (LVEDD) > 55mm;
- QRS duration ≥ 120ms;
- sinus rhythm or 1st degree heart block.

These indications may expand and be refined with the outcome of future studies. There is some evidence supporting CRT in patients in NYHA II and patients with AF. Most of the studies include patients predominantly with LBBB though it is probable that some patients with RBBB may also benefit. The aetiology of heart failure does not appear to impact on CRT's potential benefit.

## Counselling, consent, and non-responders

This is an important aspect of the management of a patient being considered for CRT. The patient should consider this therapy only with the full understanding of the facts. Expectations should not be unrealistically raised. The procedure is technically challenging and requires a high level of expertise.
- Procedural failure rate, ~ 5% (usually due to the inability to place the LV lead in an appropriate site).
- Procedural mortality, ~ 0.5%.
- Non-response rate (no clinical benefit), ~ 20–30% (not known whether this reflects patient selection, implant technique, or device programming).

## NICE guidelines for CRT

CRT is recommended as a treatment option for people with heart failure who fulfill all of the following criteria:
- NYHA III/IV
- Sinus rhythm with:
  - either QRS >150ms
  - or QRS duration 120–149ms and mechanical dyssynchrony on echocardiography
- EF ≤35%
- Optimal pharmacological therapy

Patients may be considered for an ICD (&#x1F4D5; p.190)

# Assessment of the patient for CRT

Submitting a patient to CRT requires careful assessment, investigation, and counselling.

## Timing

It is important that patients are considered for CRT at the appropriate time.

- Symptoms and disease progression stable. CRT not indicated in the patient with non-ischaemic cardiomyopathy improving with medical management.
- Post-myocardial infarction. CRT should be considered in the stable state, e.g. minimum 4 weeks post myocardial infarct.
- Post CABG. CRT should only be considered at least 3 months post-operatively.
- Stable and optimal medication. Patients should only be considered for CRT if their heart failure medication has been titrated up to the maximum tolerated dose. This does not mean that, if a patient has been intolerant of a drug or unable to take the optimal dose of a drug, they should not be considered for CRT.

## Investigations

The aim in assessing a patient for CRT is to identify the substrate for impaired LV function and address any reversible conditions. Assessment of coronary artery anatomy and/or function is essential. If surgical revascularization may lead to an improvement in LV function then this is initial management. If a patient has an alcohol-induced cardiomyopathy and continues to drink then this issue should be addressed first. The patients' symptoms and LV function should then be re-evaluated.

The following should be considered basic minimum requirements for investigations prior to CRT:

- 12 lead ECG;
- CXR;
- transthoracic echo (preferably with tissue Doppler imaging);
- coronary angiography and/or myocardial viability/ischaemia assessment:
  - myocardial perfusion scan;
  - stress echo;
  - MRI.

Objective measurements of function may be useful in assessing an individual's response to the therapy. Exercise testing (preferably with $VO_2$ measurements), 6min walk test, and quality of life questionnaire may be considered. The latter is often used as an end point in clinical studies rather than as a clinically useful tool.

**Conventional 2D echo and Doppler assessment**

It is important to a have a through assessment of cardiac function to establish possible causes for symptoms. A minimal echo data set will include the following.

- Assessment of valvular function (exclude as cause of impaired LV function).
- LV size and function:
  - LV end-diastolic and systolic dimensions;
  - LVEF;
  - interventricular septum thickness;
  - LV posterior wall thickness.
- Diastolic LV filling. Transmitral pulsed wave (PW) Doppler may demonstrate restrictive filling pattern:
  - E/A ratio > 1.5;
  - short E-wave deceleration time (< 140ms).
- Mitral regurgitation:
  - severity from colour flow and continuous wave (CW) Doppler;
  - LV contractility (dp/dt) using CW Doppler.

# Echocardiographic assessment of patients prior to CRT

Most of the large CRT studies have only used echocardiography to assess LVEF. Increasingly, echo modalities are being used to assess dyssynchrony in order to select patients for CRT. It is clear that some patients with ECG evidence of dyssynchrony (QRS > 120ms) do not have mechanical dyssynchrony. Conversely, some patients with normal QRS duration have gross dyssynchrony on echo. This section outlines techniques for assessing dyssynchrony using echocardiography. For further information see *Echocardiography*.[1]

## Classification of dyssynchrony

- AV dyssynchrony. Abnormal AV node function (1st degree block) is common in heart failure and can worsen mitral regurgitation, shorten ventricular filling time, and thus reduce LV filling.
- Interventricular dyssynchrony (Fig. 13.2). RV contraction prior to LV in the case of LBBB producing abnormal septal motion reducing LVEF.
- Intraventricular dyssynchrony (Fig. 13.2). Regions of delayed and early LV contraction contribute to increased end-systolic volume, delayed relaxation, and reduced LVEF

**Assessment of intraventricular dyssynchrony** Simple assessment can be made by measuring the difference in LV systole in M-mode of the septum (parasternal long or short axis) compared to the posterior wall. A delay of > 140ms is considered to be significant.

**Assessment of interventricular dyssynchrony** Measurements of interventricular delay can be made using PW Doppler measurements of the pulmonary artery and aortic flow. Comparison of the pre-ejection periods of the pulmonary and aortic valve openings produces a direct assessment of interventricular delay (Fig. 13.2). The pre-ejection period is defined as the time from the onset of the QRS on the surface ECG to initiation of outflow on PW Doppler. The difference between the two is considered significant if greater than 40ms.

## Reference

1 Leeson P, Mitchell A, Becher H (2007). *Echocardiography*. Oxford University Press, Oxford.

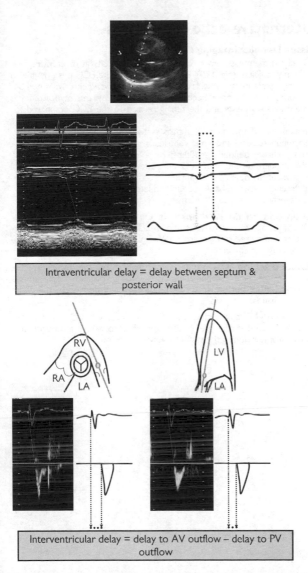

Intraventricular delay = delay between septum & posterior wall

Interventricular delay = delay to AV outflow – delay to PV outflow

**Fig. 13.2** Measurement of intraventricular and interventricular dyssynchrony. AV, Aortic valve; PV, pulmonary valve.

## Alternative echo modalities

### Tissue Doppler imaging (TDI)

TDI allows the measurement of peak systolic velocity at different regions of the myocardium (Fig. 13.3). By timing this with the ECG it is possible to precisely assess intraventricular delay and hence dyssynchrony. A number of scoring systems have been developed whereby the myocardium is divided into segments and the timing related to the ECG compared for each segment:

- maximum difference between peak systolic velocities of any 2 of 12 segments (6 basal and 6 mid ventricular segments)—intraventricular dyssynchrony defined if > 100ms;
- the standard deviation of all 12 time intervals—intraventricular dyssynchrony defined if > 33ms;
- difference between basal septum and lateral wall—intraventricular dyssynchrony defined if > 65ms.

**Strain and strain rate analysis** Off-line analysis of colour-coded TDI images allows analysis of strain, which can produce a direct assessment of the degree of myocardial deformation during systole and hence degree of dyssynchrony.

**Tissue tracking** This produces information on the LV contractile synchrony by using colour-coded displays of myocardial displacement. Regional systolic performance can be assessed and derived by the width of colour bands.

**3D imaging** More recently, 3D imaging has become available and studies have demonstrated the use of this technique to assess intraventricular dyssynchrony, including the systolic dyssynchrony index.

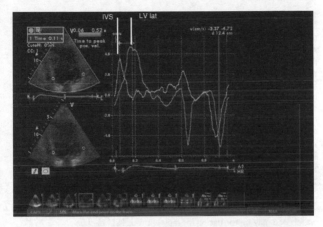

**Fig. 13.3** Tissue Doppler image of LV peak systolic velocities. Samples are taken (left images) from interventricular septum (IVS) and left ventricular lateral wall (LV lat). This demonstrates a delay of 110ms.

## Summary of dyssynchrony measurements

### Intraventricular delay

| | | |
|---|---|---|
| • M-mode | Posterior wall to septum delay | > 130ms |
| • TDI | Basal lateral wall to basal septum delay | > 100ms |
| • TDI | Maximum delay, any two segments | > 65ms |
| • TDI | Standard deviation of all 12 segments (6 basal and 6 mid ventricular) | > 33ms |

### Interventricular delay

| | | |
|---|---|---|
| • PW | Aortic valve pulmonary valve pre-ejection times | > 40ms |

# ICD or pacemaker?

Patients who are being considered for CRT have impaired LV function. A significant proportion of patients suitable for CRT will fulfil indications for an ICD. It is important to assess each patient's arrhythmic risk prior to CRT. If the patient fulfils the indications for ICD therapy then a CRT-D device should be considered. CRT-P should only be considered in those patients ineligible for ICD therapy. The evidence base to support the use of ICDs in patients in NYHA class IV is less compelling than for those in classes II and III. It is therefore conceivable that CRT-P may be considered for those with more severe heart failure (NYHA class IV) and CRT-D for those in classes II and III who are more likely to die from arrhythmias than pump failure.

Recent changes to NICE guidelines in the UK have included recommendation for implantation of ICD for patients with ischaemic heart disease, EF < 30%, no worse than NYHA class III, QRS > 120ms (Ⓜ p. 190). This therefore includes a significant number of candidates for CRT.

It is important to involve the patients in this decision process. Patient preference may be for pacing therapy without ICD backup.

# CRT in atrial fibrillation

Most clinical studies of CRT exclude patients in AF. However, AF is a common arrhythmia in patients with impaired LV function (approximately 30%). There are limited data available from sub-study analysis on the effects of CRT in AF, but patient numbers are small. These sub-studies have suggested some symptomatic benefit of CRT in patients with AF.

It is not possible to address the deleterious effects of AV dyssynchrony in patients with AF. CRT in patients with AF is also dependent on full ventricular capture. There has to be a focus, therefore, on ensuring adequate rate control to ensure minimal intrinsic ventricular activation.
- CRT device implanted (no RA lead).
- Interrogated at 4 weeks. If V pacing < 90%:
  - increase AV blocking agents;
  - consider AV node ablation.

Some operators advocate AV nodal ablation in most patients with AF for CRT to ensure biventricular pacing. If performed immediately prior to device implantation it negates the risk of lead dislodgement during a subsequent AV node ablation. The negative side is the increase in procedure time.

# Implantation techniques

## Patient preparation
Patients should be fasted pre-procedure. IV hydration should be considered, especially in patients with impaired renal function, as some patients will receive a significant contrast load during the procedure. Metformin should be stopped 48h prior to the procedure to reduce risk of lactic acidosis in response to contrast. Informed consent is essential prior to the procedure. Prophylactic IV antibiotics should be given immediately prior to the procedure, e.g. 1g flucloxacillin.

## Investigations
The following should be considered prior to the procedure:
• 12 lead ECG;
• chest X-ray;
• full blood count;
• electrolytes and serum creatinine;
• liver enzymes;
• coagulation screen.

## Laboratory/theatre setup
CRT should be performed in a fully equipped cardiac catheterization suite or operating theatre with high quality image intensifier with the ability to store acquired images. Sterile conditions and positive pressure theatre ventilation will reduce the risk of device infection.

### Laboratory/theatre checklist
The following should be readily available during the procedure:
• full resuscitation facilities—adhesive defibrillation pads should be placed on the patient at the start of the procedure;
• non-invasive blood pressure monitoring;
• arterial oxygen saturation monitor;
• IV sedation and reversal agents, analgesia;
• pericardiocentesis kit.

The 'scrub trolley' should be equipped with:
• subclavian/axillary vein cannulation equipment;
• introducer sheath and one-way valve;
• 'O' ring with side arm;
• coronary sinus cannulation catheters;
• balloon occlusion catheter;
• RA and RV pacing/ICD leads;
• LV pacing lead + stylets and/or guide wires;
• manifold and tubing connected to contrast supply and saline flush;
• local anaesthesia;
• antibiotics for pocket infiltration (e.g. gentamicin 80mg);
• sutures;
• full surgical equipment pack for device implantation.

# Implantation procedure: introduction

### Sedation and anaesthesia

- Most CRT devices are implanted using local anaesthetic and sedation.
- General anaesthesia is rarely required though it should be considered on an individual basis.

### Venous access

- Most catheters for LV lead placement are designed for the left side.
- Right-sided approaches should only be considered when venous anatomy prevents the left side from being used or when there are other anatomical reasons for not using the left, e.g. previous major trauma, infection.
- CRT-D implants should be left-sided due to the shock vector.
- The cephalic vein is rarely large enough to take all three leads so a subclavian or axillary venous approach is preferred (📖 p. 58).
- A venogram may be necessary and should be performed in the case of upgrade of an existing pacemaker/ICD.

# Right atrial and ventricular lead placement

- The RV lead is usually placed prior to  coronary sinus (CS) cannulation allowing backup RV pacing if mechanical trauma to the RBBB during attempted CS cannulation results in complete heart block.
- The RA lead can be placed either before or after CS cannulation (if placed before, may be dislodged during CS cannulation).
- Further checks of the RA and RV lead pace/sense characteristics after LV lead placement are important.
- Correct fluoroscopic appearance of all leads should be noted and documented at the end of the procedure.
- There is some evidence that placing the RV lead in the septum or RVOT rather than an apical position confers some benefit in terms of improved physiology. Acutely narrower QRS complexes and increased systolic function have been demonstrated. This may relate to more physiological RV pacing and greater separation from the LV lead.
- If a septal position is desired then an active RV lead should be used.
- Some operators advocate active leads for all cases due to the risk of dislodgement during LV lead placement.

# LV lead placement: coronary sinus cannulation

Cannulation of the CS (Fig. 13.4) provides the first challenge in placing a LV lead. Cannulation may be achieved by:
- direct cannulation of CS with introducing catheter (many different shaped catheters available);
- cannulation of the CS with a diagnostic angiographic catheter (e.g. JR4) or designed inner catheter inside the introducing catheter and then advancement of introducing catheter;
- cannulation of CS with a deflectable ablation catheter; then advancing the introducing catheter over the ablation catheter;
- some companies produce deflectable CS introducing catheters.

A number of different techniques may be used to successfully cannulate the CS. There is no single technique that can be applied to all patients as there is such a variation in CS location and direction from individual to individual. The CS ostium is often displaced from its usual position by a large dilated LV.

The following technique can be used for CS location.
- Introduce a guide catheter into the RA over a wire (PA fluoroscopy).
- Advance the catheter into the RV.
- In the LAO view, withdraw the catheter over tricuspid valve (TV) with anticlockwise torque applied.
- As catheter crosses the valve it will often displace into CS.
- The CS position can then be confirmed by advancing a wire or injection of a 'puff' of contrast into the CS.

If this fails to achieve successful cannulation the following options should be considered.
- Use different shaped introducing catheter.
- Direct catheter towards RV apex from RA and advance wire directly into CS in LAO projection.
- Inject small 'puffs' of contrast from RA to locate CS ostium.
- Introduce an angiographic catheter into the introducer catheter to provide more directionality, using the introducer catheter to offer support near proximity of the CS ostium.
- Catheters worth considering are the MP-A2, AL3, JR4, or LIMA (for more information see *Cardiac Catheterization and Coronary Angiography*).[1]

A 0.035 inch guide wire inside a diagnostic catheter within the CS guide catheter can aid insertion of the catheter into the body of the CS safely. Care should always be taken when injecting contrast or advancing catheters/guide wires, so that the end of the catheter is not directly against myocardial tissue or CS wall. This carries the risk of myocardial perforation or CS dissection.

## Reference

1 Mitchell AJ, West N, Leeson P, Banning A (2008). *Cardiac Catheterization and Coronary Angiography*, Oxford University Press, Oxford.

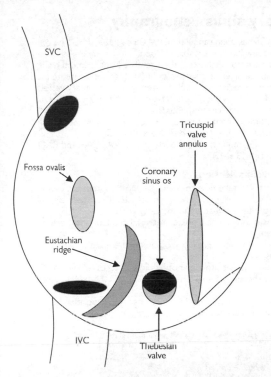

**Fig. 13.4** Schematic diagram of right atrium with anterior wall opened demonstrating CS os with its inferior border formed by the Thebesian valve (protrudes from the posterior wall of the right atrium). The Eustachian ridge is the other prominent feature that can prevent intubation of the CS os.

### The 'difficult to find' CS os

If the CS os can not be entered it is often due to the presence of a 'flap' valve over the os which needs to be 'peeled away' with the use of an inner catheter. Rotational movement of the inner catheter allows it to be advanced into the CS followed by the outer catheter.

Another technique is selective coronary angiography with a long run to watch the cardiac veins fill and empty into the CS then the RA.

## Coronary sinus venography

- Once the CS has been cannulated, the CS catheter should be gently advanced a few cm into a stable position.
- A balloon-occlusion catheter is then gently advanced into the CS.
- Care should be taken so that this catheter does not perforate the CS wall or catch in rudimentary valve tissue or small tributary vessels.
- The introducer catheter will often need withdrawing a little so that the balloon is only a few cm from CS ostium.
- A small volume of contrast should be injected prior to venography to confirm good catheter position in the central CS.
- Coronary venography is usually performed in LAO, AP, and RAO views. See Figs 13.5–13.7.

### Coronary vein selection

- It is important to take time to select the most appropriate vein.
- The target vessel will usually be the most laterally placed vein, furthest from the RV lead tip in the LAO view.
- In most cases this will be a posterolateral, lateral, or anterolateral cardiac vein.
- Venous anatomy varies greatly. Commonly there are extensive anastomoses.
- Occasionally a target site may not be directly accessible via the CS but may be through an anastomosis distally with the target vessel (Fig. 13.7).
- It is important not to place a lead in an inadequate position but to accept that the patient may require epicardial placement of a LV lead.

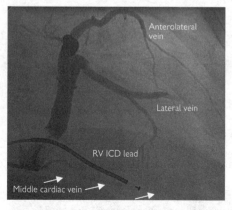

**Fig. 13.5** Coronary venogram viewed in an RAO projection (arrows point to faint middle cardiac vein originating proximal to the balloon).

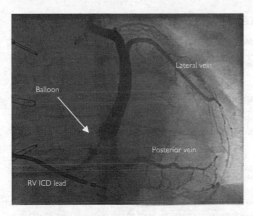

**Fig. 13.6** Coronary venogram in LAO projection. In this case there are lateral and posterior veins. The middle cardiac vein can just be seen 'ghosting' at the bottom of the image as its origin is proximal to the occlusion balloon.

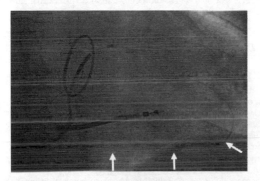

**Fig. 13.7** Guide wire demonstrating anastomosis of lateral cardiac vein with middle cardiac vein. In this case it was not possible to advance the pacing lead to a lateral position in the lateral cardiac vein, as the vessel was stenosed proximally at the point seen in the image. By advancing the lead through the middle cardiac vein the target location was achieved from the opposite direction.

# LV lead selection

Many different forms of LV lead are available. It is important to understand the particular features of each lead so that an informed decision can be made when selecting the appropriate lead. Leads can be classified as follows.

- Placement method:
  - stylet driven;
  - 'over the wire';
  - combined stylet driven and 'over the wire'.
- Electrode configuration:
  - unipolar;
  - bipolar.
- Stability configuration:
  - straight lead with barbs/anchors;
  - angulated/spiral lead;
  - lead with extendable side 'lobes'.

Each lead will have particular characteristics that will make it more suitable for a particular anatomy. For example, if there is a lateral cardiac vein in an ideal position but it is a very small vessel, then an 'over the wire' unipolar lead may be most appropriate. If, however, the target vessel is extremely large then a bipolar lead with angulated configuration or extendable side lobes might be more appropriate.

# LV lead delivery

See Fig. 13.8.

- Once the LV lead has been selected it is important to ensure maximum stability of the delivery catheter. This may require subselection of the target vein by an inner catheter. In most cases it requires placement a few cm into the coronary sinus.
- The venogram obtained in the appropriate view should be displayed during lead delivery to ensure correct placement (often the AP view is the most convenient view to use to place the LV lead).
- The lead is then delivered with the one-way return valve and 'O' ring loosened but with as little blood reflux as possible.
- The lead is screened fluoroscopically through the catheter into the CS.
- If an 'over the wire' technique is used then generally delivering the lead and wire together is preferential. It is then possible to advance the lead with a small amount of wire protruding from the end of the lead that can be used to direct it to the target vessel.
- Alternatively, the wire can be passed directly and the lead advanced over it using a 'push–pull' technique—pulling the guide wire back at the same time as advancing the lead.
- Manipulation and direction of the wire can be controlled by rotating a torque device fixed to the wire at the operator end.
- In the case of a stylet driven lead, a combination of withdrawing and advancing the stylet will allow maximum directionality.

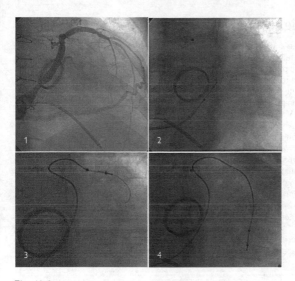

**Fig. 13.8** LV lead delivery. 1. Venography (AP) is performed first and demonstrates the target vessel to be an anterolateral cardiac vein with very little in the way of posterior or true lateral vessels. 2. An 'over the wire' lead with wire just protruding is delivered into the coronary sinus. 3. Lead steered to target vessel. 4 Wire removed once lead in target position.

# LV lead testing

- Once in place the pacing characteristics of the LV lead should be very carefully assessed.
- Basic pacing can be performed through a PSA but the device should be used to test all available configurations.
- Pacing threshold. In all possible pacing configurations:
  - unipolar/bipolar;
  - LV tip/RV ring;
  - LV ring/RV tip.
- Diaphragmatic stimulation. The output should be increased to maximum to check for diaphragmatic stimulation. If there is, then an alternate lead position should be considered. If the level at which diaphragmatic stimulation occurs is several volts greater than the pacing threshold then this may be acceptable. Remember that diaphragmatic pacing via the left phrenic nerve is often positional and may become apparent post-procedure once the patient has sat up.
- It is acceptable to have relatively high thresholds (e.g. 3.5V at 0.5ms) with LV pacing if the anatomical location is good.
- Different pulse widths should be examined as it may be possible to reduce the threshold to a lower voltage.

# Introducer catheter removal

There are many different ways to remove the introducer catheter over the LV lead. These require a degree of experience and patience so as not to displace the LV lead. The IS-1 connector prevents the catheter being pulled over lead. The LV-1 connector made by one manufacturer has a lower profile allowing the catheter to be removed over it.

- 'Slitting'. A tool may be provided to cut the catheter as it is pulled out of the venous access site. The hub of the catheter is cut first using the supplied tool. The remaining shaft of the catheter is then slit in a single movement with the cutting tool remaining in a fixed position and the catheter pulled through the cutting device. This is best done quickly without fluoroscopic imaging.
- Fixation wire. A custom designed support wire/stylet may be provided that sits in the central lumen of the lead and provides stability whilst the catheter is pulled out over the lead and then the wire.
- Lead extension. Fixes into the end of the LV lead allowing the catheter to be slid over the lead and then the extension (for LV-1 leads). Once the catheter is out the extension is removed. This is best done slowly whilst being continuously visualized fluoroscopically.

The LV lead is then usually secured in place with sutures and a cuff in the conventional manner (📖 p. 64).

## Post-implant procedure and testing

# Post-implant procedure and testing

If the device is a CRT-D then formal ventricular fibrillation (VF) induction testing will be required ( p. 230). This will usually consist of at least one VF induction with the output of the device set at 10J less than the maximum output of the device.

The following should be considered as part of the standard procedure following the implant.

- CXR: performed same day to confirm lead position and exclude complications such as pneumothorax or haemothorax.
- ECG. Confirm biventricular pacing. Failure to reduce QRS duration does not necessarily infer failure to improve dyssynchrony.
- Wound inspection.
- Pacing check: next day to confirm stable thresholds and no diaphragmatic stimulation.
- VF induction. Some centres will perform a final VF induction pre-discharge to ensure adequate safety margin for ventricular defibrillation.
- Antibiotics usually will just be given immediately prior to implantation. If the procedure has been protracted consider 5 day course of oral antibiotics.

## ECG post procedure

This is important to assess for appropriate atrial sensing and pacing (if an atrial lead has been implanted) and also for biventricular pacing. Biventricular pacing should result in a negative QRS in leads I and II and a positive QRS in V (📖 p.29).

# Complications of CRT

## Peri-implant complications

- Subclavian artery puncture (🕮 p. 86).
- Pneumothorax (1%) (🕮 p. 84).
- Pericardial tamponade (<1%) (🕮 p. 86).
- Coronary sinus dissection (1–2%): apparent with extravasation of contrast during CS cannulation or venography. In most cases there are no long-term complications but may make LV lead placement impossible. Further attempts at a later date are often successful. The patient should be monitored carefully and echocardiography performed to identify any pericardial collection.
- Coronary venous perforation (1%): apparent when the lead or guide wire is seen to advance into the pericardial space. The low pressure nature of the coronary venous system means that this often does not lead to clinically significant complications. It is important to monitor with echocardiography and regular non-invasive BP measurements.
- Complete heart block: may occur when cannulating the CS and is usually transient The RV lead should be in place and so pacing through the analyser may be used if required.
- Ventricular arrhythmias. Ventricular tachycardia may be pace terminated through the analyser or defibrillated if necessary.
- Failure to implant (up to 5%): often attempts at a later date may be successful. Alternatively, an epicardial approach should be considered. If the patient is having a CRT-D implant this should proceed with the LV port being capped with an appropriate plug to ensure continuity of the port for later attempts.
- The commonest reasons for failure to implant are:
  - failure to locate CS ostium;
  - inadequate guide catheter position;
  - poor LV venous anatomy;
  - phrenic nerve stimulation.

## Post-implant complications

- Haematoma formation. Often managed with simple pressure, in extreme cases the wound may need opening to drain and identify bleeding source(🕮 p. 88).
- Infection/sepsis (🕮 p. 90).
- Lead displacement.
- Venous occlusion and SVC syndrome may occur due to the bulk of the three leads in the venous system. If it is apparent at the time of the implant that venous flow may be compromised, anticoagulation with heparin and subsequently warfarin should be considered (🕮 p. 90).
- Thromboembolism is unusual but should be suspected if patients present with symptoms consistent with pulmonary infarction.

# CRT device programming

The basic programming of pacemaker and ICD functions remains unchanged from conventional devices. The specific issues that have to be addressed with CRT are the relative timings of pacing:
- atrioventricular (AV) delay;
- interventricular (VV) delay.

A reasonable starting point is to leave the settings at default (e.g. AV delay 100 to 120ms, LV offset 0 to −20ms). An example of a resulting ECG is demonstrated in Fig. 13.9. However, it is important to reassess the patient after a few weeks. Assessment of functional status such as exercise testing and 6 minute walk test may be useful. The device should then undergo a process of optimization. Haemodynamic response may be assessed using:
- echocardiography (most common; see *Echocardiography*);[9]
- invasive BP monitor (during implant).

In most cases this will assess different AV and VV parameters, leaving the device set up to those that give the most improvement in haemodynamic response. This does not always result in an improvement in functional status so it is important to reassess this.

## Optimization of AV delay
This can be achieved by altering the AV delay and aiming for the following.
- Increased aortic velocity time integral (stroke volume).
- Prolongation of diastolic filling: assessed using PW Doppler of transmitral blood flow. If the AV delay is too long there will be fusion of the E and A waves. Optimization of AV delay will lead to separation of E and A waves.
- Reduced mitral regurgitation (MR): assessed by colour Doppler and reduction in backward flow signal of CW Doppler of the MR.

A beneficial improvement in one parameter may have a detrimental effect on another so optimization involves achieving a balanced improvement of all parameters.

## Optimization of VV delay
Inter- and intraventricular dyssynchrony can be dramatically altered by adjusting the VV delay.
- TDI can assess mechanical delay at different myocardial segments. Alteration of the VV delay will allow an assessment of the greatest overall improvement in dyssynchrony.
- M-mode septal to posterior wall delay can be corrected by altering the VV delay. The delay that produces least delay should be considered as the optimal setting.
- Some devices can 'automatically optimize' based on timing differences in LV and RV electrograms during RV and LV pacing.

## Reference
9 Leeson P, Mitchell A, Becher H (2007). *Echocardiography*. Oxford University Press, Oxford.

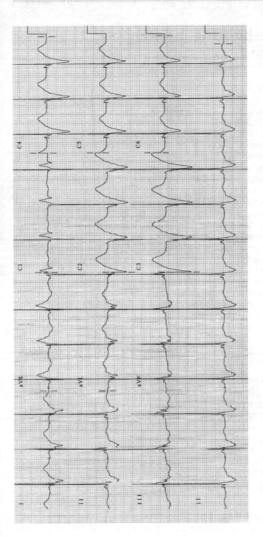

**Fig. 13.9** ECG recorded post-CRT implant. Note small bipolar pacing stimulus pr or to P wave followed by further small bipolar stimulus prior to QRS complex. For RV pacing, then 80 ms into the QRS complex the unipolar stimulus from the LV lead is seen. Often the LV stimulus is not cistinguished from RV as the default setting on most devices is with no delay.

# Troubleshooting in CRT

CRT is an evolving therapy and remains complex in terms of patient selection, device implantation, and follow-up.

## Device-related complications

- Standard device-related complications, e.g. pneumothorax, infection, haematoma, should be managed in the usual manner.
- LV lead displacement. There is an increased risk of LV lead displacement compared to RA and RV leads.
  - Displacement may occur early or late and occasionally this may be months post-implantation reflecting the relative paucity of fibrosis formation compared to that with RA/RV leads.
  - Invariably LV lead displacement requires complete repositioning of the lead with cannulation of the CS with a guide catheter.
  - Occasionally with minimal displacement, use of a stylet or guide wire may be sufficient to reposition the lead.
  - It is important to understand why the lead has moved so as not to have further lead displacement.
  - In some circumstances switching to a different lead that may be more suited to longer-term stability in the specific vein may be required, e.g. a larger lead.
- Phrenic nerve stimulation: this can be difficult to rectify.
  - It is possible to get no stimulation at the time of implant but to get stimulation of the diaphragm when the patient is upright.
  - The threshold at which diaphragmatic stimulation is seen should be recorded.
  - Provided there is sufficient difference from the LV pacing threshold, simple programming of the LV output may resolve the issue. If not, the lead will require repositioning.

## Non-responders

This remains one of the greatest challenges of CRT with non-response rates in the region of 20–30%. The reason for non-response is likely to be one of the following.

- Lack of mechanical dyssynchrony. Some patients with broad QRS complexes do not have mechanical dyssynchrony. Most of the large studies did not exclude these patients.
- Suboptimal lead placement. In the case of non-response but suitable alternate target vessels, lead repositioning may be recommended.
- Device setup incorrect. Optimization of AV and VV delay should be very carefully assessed.

## Pharmacological review

It is important to review all medication soon after CRT (within 2 weeks) as some patients make a dramatic acute haemodynamic improvement with CRT. This can lead to a reduction in diuretic requirement.

## Long-term follow-up

## Long-term follow-up

Patients with CRT devices will require long-term follow-up of both their device and their heart failure. In the case of CRT-D this is most likely at a frequency of 3 or 6 months when stable and, with CRT-P, 6 or 12 months. It is important that the pharmacological aspect of their management is consistently reviewed and optimized.

In the event of deterioration of heart failure the following should be considered.

- Progression of primary cause of heart failure: important to consider re-evaluation of reversible substrates and optimization of heart failure treatment.
- Failure of CRT: assess LV pacing to ensure no increase in threshold and consider repeat echo optimization of device settings. Review AV interval to ensure that intrinsic ventricular activation is not inhibiting CRT. Displacement rates of 10% at 6 months have been observed.

# Future developments in CRT

CRT continues to evolve and it is likely that there will be several significant advances in the therapy in the near future.

- Remote device follow-up.
  - Systems are available that allow devices to be interrogated in the patient's home.
  - This is performed using wireless technologies that allow interface with a device in the patient's home that can then transtelephonically transmit the data to the physician.
  - This has the potential to allow regular, even daily, device interrogation and allow for earlier troubleshooting.
- Physiological data.
  - Increasing data are becoming available on the trends in patients physiology, e.g. heart rate variability, activity, etc.
  - These data can be used to assess the impact of CRT and allow for optimizing in an individual.
  - Some devices measure transthoracic impedance to give a correlate of pulmonary oedema. This has the potential to alert the patient and physician if there is a trend towards pulmonary oedema.
  - Decreases in impedance appear to occur up to 2 weeks prior to hospitalization for heart failure.
- Haemodynamic sensors. Ultimately it might be possible to have a direct assessment of the patient's measured arterial pressure or cardiac output.
- Refinement of indications.
  - It is likely that some patients with narrow QRS complexes but dyssynchrony may benefit from CRT and also some patients with broad complexes may not benefit.
  - Understanding this may improve the non-response rate.
  - CRT appears to offer some benefit to those patients with congenital heart disease who may have RBBB but impaired ventricular function.
  - There are some groups of patients who require further prospective data to identify the role of CRT. These groups include those with atrial fibrillation and patients with conventional indications for pacing and poor LV function.

# System and lead extractions

# General principles

With the rising prevalence of implantable pacemakers and defibrillators, the need for explants or extractions of transvenous leads has recently increased.

- *Explant* is defined as the removal of a lead that has been implanted for less than 1 year.
- *Extraction* refers to the removal of a lead that has been implanted for more than 1 year.

The goal is to completely remove all components of transvenous leads without complications. The major hurdle to extraction is fixation of the lead by fibrous tissue to the venous system or endocardium. Completely successful extraction may be accomplished in 95%, partial extraction in 3%, and failure in 2%.

# Indications

The decision to explant or extract leads should be based on the principle that the risk of the procedure should be less than the risk of leads or devices remaining in place.

### Infection-related indications

- Endocarditis with lead involvement.
- Recurrent pocket infection.
- Pocket erosion or perforation.

### Lead-related indications

- Retained lead causing serious arrhythmias, thrombosis, or physical threat.
- Venous obstruction with need to implant new system.
- Lead interactions.
- Lead fracture or failure.
- Ineffective therapy (high pacing or defibrillation thresholds).

### Patient-related indications

- Resolution of arrhythmic risk (e.g. viral cardiomyopathy).
- Intractable pain syndrome (a rare cause but may be necessary).

**Extraction for infection**

If an extraction is being performed for infection it is important to image the leads to assess for vegetations. Retrospective data have shown that percutaneous removal of leads with vegetations larger than 1cm is associated with a significant risk of pulmonary embolism. Therefore, TOE is recommended to define the size of any vegetations. Vegetations >1cm in size indicate surgical removal through an open-chest approach is appropriate.

# Patient preparation

## Prior to procedure

- History and examination:
  - original implant indication;
  - previous procedural details including difficulties encountered and venous access sites, active or passive fixation leads, any redundant leads, subcutaneous or subpectoral pocket;
  - comorbidities.
- Investigations:
  - FBC;
  - U & E;
  - clotting screen;
  - ESR, CRP, blood cultures;
  - group and save;
  - 12 lead ECG;
  - CXR: overpenetrated PA and lateral views;
  - Echocardiography: transthoracic and transoesophageal (if endocarditis suspected).
- Interrogation of the pacemaker or ICD: assess pacing and sensing thresholds; assess pacing dependency (if pacing dependent will require temporary pacing through the procedure).
- Preparation for general anaesthesia (for leads implanted > 6 months): to minimize patient discomfort and optimize haemodynamics.
- Consent. Patients need to fully informed of risk including mortality with lead extraction (see complications 📖 p. 330).

## In the pacing laboratory

- General and local anaesthesia (due to the discomfort related to extraction general anaesthesia is recommended for all cases).
- Peripheral IV access.
- Peripheral arterial access and pressure monitoring.
- 3 Lead ECG monitoring.
- High-magnification fluoroscopy.
- Temporary pacing equipment.
  - Temporary pacing is required prior to extraction for a patient who is pacing-dependent—usually via femoral vein.
- Echocardiography.
- Pericardiocentesis equipment.
- Access to surgical backup should be established.

# Tools for extraction

Specific tools have been designed for lead extraction and should be used in every case. A relatively simple case may easily be complicated if the correct approach is not adopted.

**Lead cutter** Specialized heavy-duty scissors designed to cleanly cut lead insulations and coils to prevent retraction of inner lead conductor.

**Coil expander** This conical expander is used to enlarge the often crushed proximal end of the inner conductor after cutting to allow proper sizing of locking stylets.

## Locking stylet
- This stylet is advanced down the lumen of the inner coil to the distal end.
- When deployed, the stylet expands and 'locks' within the lumen.
- It allows traction pressure to be transmitted down to the lead tip and prevents lead breakage.
- A modern locking stylet expands throughout the length of the lead and can be reversible and reusable.

## Extraction sheaths
- These may be metallic (e.g. steel) but more commonly polymeric (e.g. Teflon).
- An inner sheath telescopes over the lead to shear away adhering fibrosis. This is achieved by pressure, radiofrequency energy (electrosurgical-dissection sheaths; EDS) or laser (Excimer system). Their success rates are comparable.
- An outer sheath telescopes over the inner sheath to provide support and prevent kinking during extraction. At the level of endocardium, it allows for counter-traction.
- Following extraction, sheath allows venous access if a new pacing systems is to be implanted.

## Systems for extraction (Fig. 14.1)

### EDS system
- This involves electrodiathermy between two electrodes at the tip of the extraction sheath.
- Preferred for leads with shorter implant durations.
- Less expensive than laser system.
- Less likely to cause vascular damage.

### Laser system
- The laser extraction sheaths significantly reduce the pressure required to dissect through fibrotic tissue.
- Best for extracting multiple leads or old leads and in occluded veins.
- Circumferential cutting may damage SVC.

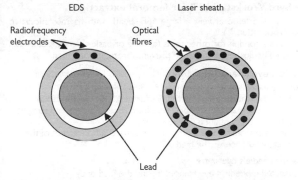

**Fig. 14.1** Tips of an EDS and a laser extraction sheath. The EDS sheath tip is bevelled with the electrodes at the leading edge, allowing for these to be placed on the inner side when turning tight corners, e.g. bending into the SVC.

## The Byrd Workstation™ for femoral extraction

Insert into the femoral vein a large 16F sheath with haemostatic valve (Byrd Workstation™).

- It acts as a conduit for other tools (a snare or basket) to extract leads.
- It should be flushed regularly to prevent thrombus formation.

## Needle's eye snare (Fig. 14.2)

- Complete extraction: success rate 85–90%.
- Useful if the lead to be extracted has formed a loop in the atrium.
- Two components: hook-shaped wire loop (needle's eye), and straight wire (threader) contained in a 12F sheath.
- Advancement of threader completes the snare; advancement of the inner catheter secures the lead.

*Using the needle's eye snare*

- Advance the needle's eye to hook round the lead body.
- Advance the threader to trap the lead.
- Advance the sheath over the snare to grasp the lead.
- Pull back the needle's eye, threader, and sheath together to prolapse into the workstation.
- The workstation may be advanced up to the endocardium for counter-traction.

## Amplatz goose-neck snare and deflecting wire

- Place both snare and wire in the atrium or IVC via the workstation.
- The deflector wire is used to catch the lead first.
- The snare is advanced to grasp the deflecting wire tip and to loop round the lead body.
- Extract lead as for needle's eye snare.

## Helical loop basket (Fig 14.3)

This is used in a similar manner to the goose-neck snare.

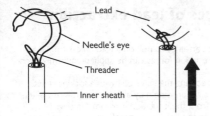

**Fig. 14.2** The needle's eye snare. Advancing the inner sheath pulls the lead to the sheath.

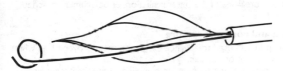

**Fig. 14.3** Helical loop basket with tip-deflecting wire.

# Basic techniques of lead extraction

## Lead control

- The operator should not attempt to pull on a lead unless total lead control is achieved and traction forces can be applied uniformly over the entire length of the lead.
- Control is achieved by securing the inner coil with a locking stylet. In addition, the outer insulation is held by a tie so that the risk of inner conductor detachment from the insulation is minimized (Fig. 14.4). This tie is then secured to the loop on the locking stylet on which traction can be applied.
- When traction is applied, the tensile properties of the lead should be constantly assessed. Changes in the tensile response may indicate detachment of the lead from fibrotic tissue, unravelling of the inner conductor, breakage of the outer insulation, or detachment of stylet from lead.

## Pressure and counterpressure

This is the principle used to advance extraction sheaths over a lead whilst maintaining tension of the lead.

- Pressure describes the pushing force applied to the sheaths that is directed towards the heart.
- Counterpressure refers to the pulling force applied to the lead in the opposite direction.
- Disruption of fibrosis is achieved by balanced and steady pressure and counterpressure applied tangentially to the vessel wall.
- Excessive pressure on the sheaths may perforate vessel wall of SVC or myocardium.
- Excessive counterpressure on the lead may lacerate vessel wall or avulse myocardium.

## Traction and countertraction (Fig. 14.5)

This is the principle used when the extraction lead is at the endocardium at the tip of the lead.

- Traction refers to the pulling force applied on the lead with or without an overlying extraction sheath.
- Countertraction is applied when traction on the lead is opposed by pushing pressure of the overlying sheath on to the endocardium to limit myocardial invagination or avulsion.

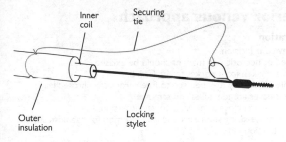

**Fig. 14.4** Locking stylet and securing tie.

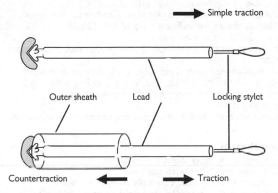

**Fig. 14.5** Traction and countertraction.

# Superior venous approach

## Preparation
- Subclavicular incision.
- Infected or necrotic skin margins should be excised.
- Swabs are taken from pocket for M, C, & S.
- Unipolar diathermy may be used to free chronically fibrosed leads.
- Suture sleeves are identified and removed.
- Expose leads as close as possible to vein insertion.
- Prepare purse-string suture around lead insertion for haemostasis after extraction.

## Lead
- Identify leads using the serial numbers.
- An active lead should be unscrewed prior to cutting.
- Use cutting scissors to cut lead as far as possible from vein insertion.
- Use scalpel to circumferentially cut away 10mm of insulation at the proximal end of the lead if necessary.
- Use a coil expander (spike like tool) to enlarge the lumen of the inner conductor.
- A standard pacemaker stylet is passed to the lead tip to clear debris.
- Pass locking stylet to the lead tip. The tip of the locking stylet may be radio-opaque; thus insertion may be guided by fluoroscopy.
- Deploy locking stylet.
- Secure proximal outer insulation using strong suture and tie to loop in the locking stylet.

## Extraction sheaths
- Size according to the outer diameter of the lead.
- Flush all sheaths with heparinized saline.
- Metallic sheaths (if used) should be replaced by more flexible polymeric sheaths after access to the subclavian vein to avoid SVC perforation.
- Laser sheaths will need to be calibrated before use. Protective glasses are to be worn.
- Insert sheaths over lead and advance into venous system under fluoroscopy.
- Slow, steady, and balanced pressure and counterpressure should be applied if fibrosis is encountered, maintaining sheath angle parallel to the lead.
- Outer sheath is then advanced on to the endocardial surface for countertraction.
- EDS electrodes should be kept on the inner curve of the lead during advancement into the SVC to prevent SVC perforation (remembering the electrodes are on the leading edge of the bevel). Significant rotational torque may need to be applied to the sheath.
- Once the inner sheath is within the cardiac silhouette, radiofrequency or laser energy should not be applied further to avoid myocardial perforation.

# Femoral venous approach

Insert the Byrd Workstation™ (use contralateral side to temporary wire if used).

### The needle's eye snare
- Advance the needle's eye to hook round the lead body.
- Advance the threader to trap the lead.
- Advance the sheath over the snare to grasp the lead.
- Pull back the needle's eye, threader, and sheath together to prolapse into the workstation.
- The workstation may be advanced up to the endocardium for counter-traction.

### Amplatz goose-neck snare or helical loop basket and tip-deflecting wire
- Useful for larger leads and for leads with proximal free ends in the right atrium or IVC.
- The guide wire loops around the lead and is grasped by the snare.

### Tips
- The lead may stretch or break because of no locking stylets and multiple retrievals may be required.
- If the lead will not prolapse into workstation, the lead, snare, and workstation may have to be retracted and removed in one unit.
- After removal of all extraction devices, prolonged pressure (over 10min) over the venepuncture site is necessary for haemostasis.

# Defibrillator and coronary sinus lead extractions

### ICD lead extraction
- This is more complicated and prolonged than pacemaker lead extraction because:
  - diameter of ICD lead is larger;
  - multiple conductors increase the rate of mechanical failure;
  - defibrillator coils stimulate more fibrosis.
- The same tools and techniques are used as those described for pacing lead extraction.
- If present a separate SVC coil lead should be removed first because it is shorter and may disrupt SVC fibrosis, making subsequent RV lead extraction easier.
- In experienced hands, successful complete removal can be achieved in > 95%.

### CS lead extraction
- Limited experience reported in small series, but it appears to be safe.
- Simple traction of lead is often successful.
- Powered sheaths may be required to free fibrosis in subclavian veins and SVC.
- Laser extraction in the CS is feasible, but its safety is not yet established.
- Transfemoral approach may be helpful if fibrotic attachment of CS leads to other leads.

# Open surgical lead extraction

### Indications
- Failed percutaneous lead extraction.
- Surgical cardiac disease.
- Endocarditis with large vegetations (> 1cm).

### Procedure
- Standard midline thoracotomy or lateral thoracotomy with minimal atriotomy.
- Increased morbidity and longer recovery time compared with intravascular approach.
- Reported mortality rates are variable: 0–12.5%.

# Post lead extraction

### Re-implantation
- In the absence of infection, re-implantation of new endocardial leads is possible by the retained guide wire technique using the extraction sheaths as a conduit (📖 p. 58).
- Long introducers may help to bypass torn or stenotic venous structures.
- New leads should have active fixation and be implanted away from extracted sites to avoid fibrotic endocardium.
- In the presence of infection, re-implantation is delayed for antibiotic therapy. If patient is pacing-dependent a tunnelled temporary system may be implanted until infection is eradicated and a new system is implanted. Microbiological advice should be sought regarding duration of therapy.
- Re-implant device only after resolution of infection and normalization of inflammatory markers.

### Post-procedural care
- Pain control.
- Wound haemostasis.
- CXR (exclude pneumothorax and haemothorax).
- Echocardiography.

# Complications

Lead extractions are risky procedures. The risk of death and potentially life-threatening complications in the Cook Extraction Registry were 0.6% and 2.5%, respectively. With experience, high volume operators have reported figures of 0.04% and 1.4%, respectively. Hence lead extractions should only be performed by or supervised by an experienced operator with the appropriate tools. Adequate facilities for haemodynamic monitoring and treatment of potential complications should be in place.

### Factors associated with increased risk of complications
- Female.
- Longer duration of implant.
- Multiple leads.
- Experience of the operator (< 50 cases).

### Major complications
- Overall, 1–2%.
- Myocardial avulsion.
- Cardiac tamponade.
- SVC or subclavian vascular tear.
- Pneumothorax.
- Pulmonary embolism.
- Death.

**Minor complications**
- Haematoma.
- Venous thrombosis.
- Cardiac arrhythmias.
- Retained lead fragments.

# Device clinic and follow-up

# The device clinic

### Facilities
In order to assess patients safely and in privacy a dedicated area is required along with the following:
- full resuscitation equipment;
- technical files for all patients;
- programmers for all appropriate devices;
- 12 lead ECG;
- medical grade pacemaker magnet;
- facility for emergency patient admission;
- access to radiography department (for CXR if required);
- computer access to database to store patient information.

### Device follow-up schedule
The follow-up schedule for a device (new implant or pulse generator replacement) is usually as follows.
- First visit: 6 weeks post implant
- Maintenance: 6–12 month intervals (6 month for ICD).
- Approaching ERI/EOL: 2–3 month intervals.

Patients with a CRT device may be seen at 3–6 month intervals depending mainly on their clinical status.

### Patient review
*History*
It is important to obtain a history to identify clinical or pacemaker-related problems. Specifically the following enquiries are important.
- Chest pain. Pericarditic chest pain may occur following perforation of the myocardium by pacing lead (⬚ p. 86). Cardiac ischaemia may be worsened with aggressive rate response algorithms.
- Syncope. Devices can record EGM related to high atrial and ventricular rates. Correlation of these with a syncopal episode may aid diagnosis. Alternatively, syncope with no evidence of abnormal rhythm may suggest an alternative cause (e.g. epilepsy) or, with neurocardiogenic syncope, that the vasomotor component is more important than cardioinhibitory. Device malfunction with loss of capture or oversensing with underpacing due to lead fracture or EMI can also lead to syncope.
- Palpitations. EGM recording can again correlate symptoms with arrhythmias that may require therapy on their own merit, e.g. SVT, AF.
- Dyspnoea and fatigue. Loss of LV capture, pacemaker syndrome, sustained tachyarrhythmias, loss of pacing in a patient with low underlying rate can all cause dyspnoea.
- Medication review.

*Examination*
- Wound. This is important not only at the first follow-up but at all visits as problems can occur later including threatened erosion, infection, and generator migration necessitating operative intervention.

**Rationale for device follow-up**

- The first visit allows for an initial assessment to confirm wound healing and recovery from the procedure. Lead parameters and programming functions can also be checked to ensure they are correctly set.
- The main reason for subsequent visits is to assess the battery and lead parameters in order to organize for timely pulse generator replacement and identify any developing problem with the leads.
- The device clinic is also an opportunity to pick up changes in a patient's symptoms that warrant further medical review or alteration in pacing settings. This is particularly important for ICD and CRT clinics where patients often are also being treated for heart failure.
- Finally, the stored EGMs and records of mode-switch episodes, AF burden, or device therapy may be useful in decisions about changes in treatment.

# Pacemaker follow-up

## Pacemaker testing

The correct programmer with appropriate software should be used to interrogate the pacemaker. The following is the minimum information to record at follow-up:
- impedance of pacing lead(s);
- sensed R ± P wave amplitude;
- pacing threshold in RV ± RA lead (autocapture for RV on new devices);
- battery voltage and impedance (manufacturers will have specific ERI levels).

## Other interrogated information

Increasingly, complex pacemakers give more information that may be of use to the physician as an aid to management, diagnosis, and optimization of programming. The information available depends on the pacemaker type but basic information available on most devices is as follows.
- Event counters:
  - percentage sensed and paced events in the atrium and ventricle (these may be displayed as histograms showing percentage at different rates; see Fig. 15.1);
  - atrial/ventricular tachycardias;
  - AF burden;
  - mode-switching episodes (📖 p. 112);
  - rate drop response episodes (📖 p. 118);
  - pacemaker-mediated tachycardias (📖 p. 128);
  - patient activity (📖 p. 124).
- Stored EGMs:
  - atrial arrhythmias;
  - ventricular arrhythmias.

## Recorded information

As well as the interrogated information, the basic programming and any changes to this should be recorded including:
- pacing rates;
- pacing mode;
- underlying rhythm (record if not able to record at slowest rate programmable on the pacemaker);
- programmed lead outputs;
- programmed lead sensitivities;
- programmed A/V delay.

At the end of any interrogation make sure that, once all information is recorded, final programming printouts are made and stored electronically (usually on a disk or hard-drive within the programmers) and the counters are reset. The patient will also need a new appointment according to the standard follow-up procedures or based on what has been found during the clinic.

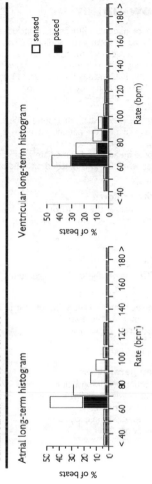

**Fig. 15.1** Atrial and ventricular event histograms.

# ICD follow-up

The follow-up of patients with an ICD includes all of the information obtained for a pacemaker with additional components. A number of patients will have received therapies and so may have questions and concerns regarding this. This, in combination with the extra information required from the ICD, means these patients require more time in clinic. The additional information required is as follows.

### Battery voltage
- Most modern devices reach ERI around 2.45–2.55V.
- Some devices will alert the patient when ERI is reached with a beep or vibration.
- Patients should be admitted immediately for generator replacement if it is unclear when ERI was reached or if the battery is at the end of life (EOL).

### Auto capacitor reform
- Automatically charges the capacitors every 1–6 months.
- Another indicator for generator replacement if the charge time is extended.

### ICD lead
- Shock impedance.
- Real-time EGM recordings in all configurations including shock coils.

### Event logs
These will give information on episodes of ventricular arrhythmias including:
- numbers of non-sustained episodes;
- therapies delivered in each zone;
- outcome of therapies;
- electrogram recordings.

### Programmed parameters
As well as recording the information required for a pacemaker, additional information that needs recording includes:
- programmed detection zones;
- programmed therapies in each zone;
- bradycardia pacing.

# CRT follow-up

In addition to the appropriate pacemaker checks the information for CRT follow up is as follows (see Fig. 15.2).

## LV lead
- Threshold.
- New devices are now available that can assess the LV threshold on a daily basis and set the output of the LV lead appropriately.

## Percentage biventricular paced
- The percentage of biventricular pacing is important and should be maintained at > 80%.
- If it falls below this in a patient with AF and increasing AV nodal blocking agents does not improve the figure, AV nodal ablation should be considered.
- If the figure is < 80% in sinus rhythm the AV delay may need reprogramming appropriately.

## Clinical reviews and medications
It is very important to assess medications at follow-up as the improvements in haemodynamics with CRT may lead to a reduction in the need for diuretics.

| Patient sticker: | Device: | Implant date: | |
|---|---|---|---|
| Date | | | |
| Battery voltage | | | |
| Last charge time + date | | | |
| Autocap (months) | | | |
| P wave | | | |
| R wave (RV) | | | |
| R wave (LV) | | | |
| Atrial threshold | | | |
| RV threshold | | | |
| LV threshold | | | |
| Atrial impedance | | | |
| RV impedance | | | |
| LV impedance | | | |
| Shock/HVB | | | |
| Medical Rx change | Yes /No | Yes/No | Yes/No |
| | | | |
| VF episodes | | | |
| Outcomes | | | |
| FVT episodes | | | |
| Outcomes | | | |
| VT/VT-1 episodes | | | |
| Outcomes | | | |
| Other episodes e.g. NSVT, M/S | | | |
| | | | |
| VF detection | | | |
| VF therapy | | | |
| FVT detection | | | |
| FVT therapy | | | |
| VT detection | | | |
| VT therapy | | | |
| | | | |
| Sensitivity (A & V) | | | |
| Pacing mode & rate | | | |
| Wound check | Yes/No | Yes/No | Yes/No |
| Reprogramme settings | Yes/No | Yes/No | Yes/No |
| Disk save/counters cleared | Yes/No | Yes/No | Yes/No |
| Next F/Up | | | |
| Cardiac physiologist | | | |
| Comments | | | |

**Fig. 15.2** Example of reporting form for a CRT-D follow up.

# Lifestyle issues, patients' concerns, and devices

# Post-implant advice

Following a device implant patient education is essential. Patients for all devices should be advised of the following.

- Always carry device identification card.
- Keep wound dry for 5–7 days.
- Stitch removal (if non-absorbable skin suture) at 7–10 days.
- Avoid abducting ipsilateral arm higher than horizontal and avoid vigorous activity of this arm for 2–4 weeks.
- Driving regulations as appropriate.
- Advised to attend if signs of fever, infection, pain, or erythema at wound site.
- Routine follow-up following implant at 6 weeks; then annual for pacemaker and 6 monthly for ICD.
- Point of contact for problems and, for ICD, what to do in the event of a shock.

# Driving regulations and devices

Fitness to drive regulations in the UK are drawn up by the Secretary of State's Honorary Medical Advisory Panels. A group 1 license includes cars and motor cycles. A group 2 license includes large lorries and buses. These are updated every 6 months and the information that follows is only accurate at the time of writing. Up to date information from the DVLA is available at: *http://www.dvla.gov.uk/media/pdf/medical/aagv1.pdf*

## UK driving regulations and pacemakers

It is important that patients are informed about driving regulations, which are relatively simple for permanent pacemakers. There are specific regulations for the underlying rhythm disturbances and conditions (syncope, heart block) for which a device is to be implanted. Patients should be informed appropriately whilst awaiting an implant and the current DVLA guidelines should be consulted.

### Summary of current UK driving regulations regarding permanent pacemakers

|  | Group 1 license | Group 2 license |
|---|---|---|
| Primary implant | Driving must cease for 1 week. Driving may be permitted thereafter provided there is no other disqualifying condition. *DVLA need not be notified* | Disqualifies for 6 weeks. Re/licensing may be permitted thereafter provided there is no other disqualifying condition |
| Box change | As for primary implant | As for primary implant |

## UK driving regulations and ICDs

Compared to regulations regarding permanent pacemakers, those surrounding ICDs are more complicated. An ICD, however, is a permanent bar to a group 2 license and all further discussion concerns a group 1 license.

Following an ICD implant for a sustained ventricular arrhythmia the patient should not drive in the following settings:
• 6 months post-implant;
• 6 months after any appropriate shock or symptomatic ATP;
• 2 years after any appropriate incapacitating therapy, e.g. loss of consciousness (6 months if steps taken to prevent recurrence and absence of further symptoms);
• following inappropriate shock, 1 month after cause completely controlled;
• 1 month after any lead revision or change in anti-arrhythmic drugs;
• 1 week after box change.

Resumption of driving requires that:
• the device is subject to regular review with interrogation;
• there is no other disqualifying condition.

For patients presenting with a non-disqualifying event, e.g. haemodynamically stable, non-incapacitating VT, the patient can drive 1 month after implant if all of the following are met:
- LVEF > 35%;
- no fast VT at EPS (RR interval < 250ms);
- any VT induced/terminated by ATP twice during post-implant EPS.

For patients at high risk of ventricular arrhythmia with a prophylactic ICD following implant:
- patient not to drive for 1 month;
- should therapy be delivered usual criteria apply and DVLA should be notified.

# Frequently asked questions

The following is general advice for patients. The word device refers to either a pacemaker or ICD.

### Can I use a cellular phone?

Yes. Modern devices are designed to resist interference from mobile devices.

- Keep the mobile phone 15cm away from the device, hold the phone to the opposite ear, and do not keep the phone in the ipsilateral breast pocket.

### Are household appliances safe?

Yes. This includes: microwave ovens; electric blankets; stereos; hair dryers; electric shavers; vacuum cleaners.

- The following should be kept 15cm away from the device: magnets; large stereo speakers; handheld massagers.

### Can I use power tools?

Some. If at any point whilst using a tool you become dizzy, faint, or aware of a rapid heartbeat move further away from the tool (any potential effects will be transient).

- For mains-powered tools plugged into the mains (e.g. electric drills and sanders) and battery powered tools (e.g. cordless screwdrivers) keep the motor at least 15cm away from the device.
- For petrol-powered tools (e.g. lawn mowers, leaf blowers) keep the motor part 30cm away from the device. Do not work on the tool when it is running and do not touch the coil, distributor, or spark plug cables whilst it is running.
- Avoid using chainsaws and welding. The ignition systems of petrol powered chainsaws produce electromagnetic energy that can lead to inappropriate pacing or a shock from an ICD. Electric chainsaws pose less of a risk but should still be avoided. Loss of consciousness using a chainsaw could lead to significant injury. The electromagnetic energy generated from different types of welding is variable and it is recommended to avoid all forms. Welding can lead to inappropriate pacing from the device or inhibition of pacing.

### Can I work on my car?

Avoid working near the distributor and spark plug cables on a running car. Any alteration to the distributor should be done with the engine off.

### Can I have X-rays, CT, or ultrasound scans?

Yes. These are safe with a device implanted.

### Can I have an MRI scan?

No. Current advice is that you should not as the MRI scan could alter the function of your device and also lead to heating of the lead tip potentially leading to loss of pacing.

### Are medical procedures safe?

Most procedures are safe with a device implanted. Some procedures such as lithotripsy, diathermy, radiation therapy, and electrosurgery produce electromechanical interference. Discussion with your consultant before undergoing such procedures is advised.

### Can I play sports?

Yes, however contact sports, e.g. karate, rugby, are not advised due to the risk of damage to the device.

### Can I travel?

Yes. Most patients with a device can travel without any limitations. Support for devices is available in most countries.

### Can I go through airport security detectors?

Although going through these devices is unlikely to affect your device it will set off the alarm due to the metal housing. You are therefore advised to show your device identity card and to undergo alternative security checks such as a hand-held security wand (which should be kept away from your device) or a hand search. With an ICD ask for a hand search as a security wand may lead to shock.

### Can I go through shop antitheft detectors?

Yes. However, these do develop electromagnetic interference and so you should walk through at a normal pace and not stand still near the detection equipment.

### If I get a shock from my ICD whilst holding my partner will it hurt them?

No. They may feel you have muscle spasm during the shock, which may be startling but it will not hurt.

# Actions in the event of a shock from an ICD

Patients will most likely have been unaware of any discomfort during DFTs at the time of implant or subsequently due to sedation or general anaesthetic. Patients should be made aware of what to do in the event of a shock and a plan will help in what can be a very traumatic time, especially for a first shock.

Patients should have a point of contact, e.g. ICD nurse specialist, whom they can contact in such an event or for general advice.

Urgent admission for a single shock is not required. The patient should attend for interrogation as soon as it is reasonable to assess (patient should not drive until they have been assessed). In the event of a shock the following may be required and the patient advised accordingly.

- Diagnosis of the appropriateness of the shock (e.g. inappropriate shock due to AF).
- 'Phantom' shock (patients felt a shock but no recorded shock delivered by the device).
- Change in medical management, e.g. increase in beta blockers.
- Advice regarding driving (restrictions may apply).
- Need for admission (e.g. lead fracture leading to oversensing off noise requiring operative intervention).
- Reassurance.

If the patient receives multiple shocks they should go immediately to hospital as it may be an 'electrical storm' with recurrent ventricular arrythmias, a lead malfunction leading to inappropriate shocks, or supraventricular arrythmias.

# Perioperative management of devices

# General principles

Expanding use of pacemakers and ICDs has made it common for patients with devices to present for elective or emergency surgery and other interventional procedures.

The key issue in perioperative management is the potential for electromagnetic interference (EMI) altering performance of devices, possibly leading to malfunction and/or adverse clinical consequences.

The major source of EMI is surgical electrocautery (diathermy) used for cutting and thermocoagulation. Other sources include radiofrequency current for catheter ablation, defibrillation/cardioversion, and therapeutic ionizing radiation. It is important to minimize the risk of malfunction in patients undergoing such procedures.

The American College of Cardiology (ACC)/American Heart Association (AHA) and the UK Medicines and Healthcare Products Regulatory Agency (MHRA) have recently proposed practical guidelines for perioperative management. Whilst acknowledging the risks, it should be stressed that major technological advances (titanium casing, protective circuitry, bandpass filters, noise reversion/back-up pacing modes, etc.) have markedly reduced the susceptibility of modern devices to EMI and serious events are rare.

Modern implanted devices have been engineered for a high degree of tolerance to common environmental sources of EMI. Therefore problems will only arise if there is exposure to a nearby field with a high energy level and/or frequency close to the clinical range of heart rates.

Certain factors increase susceptibility to EMI including:
• unipolar rather than bipolar leads;
• monopolar rather than bipolar diathermy (high power for cutting);
• surgical procedures in the vicinity of the device.

## Possible effects of EMI on ICDs and pacemakers

- Pacemakers may be temporarily or, rarely, permanently reset to back-up or noise-reversion mode (typically asynchronous VOO competing with underlying sinus rhythm or replacing DDD mode with loss of AV synchrony and the potential for haemodynamic deterioration).
- Temporary loss of pacemaker output due to oversensing resulting in bradycardia or asystole in pacing-dependent patients.
- Increased pacing rate due to activation of impedance-based rate-responsive sensors (pacemakers or ICDs) or inappropriate 'atrial-tracking' of the extrinsic electrical activity.
- Misclassification of electrical noise as VT or VF by ICDs, resulting in inappropriate therapies—both anti-tachycardia pacing and shocks.
- Thermal myocardial injury at the lead tip resulting in temporary or sustained dysfunction with elevated pacing thresholds, loss of capture, and/or sensing (most likely as a result of high-energy EMI such as external defibrillation).
- Permanent damage to the pulse generator circuitry of the pacemaker or ICD with malfunction or even total failure (very rare with modern devices).

# Role of magnets

In the past, magnets (Fig. 17.1) were commonly used in pacemaker patients to induce asynchronous pacing (VOO or DOO) during electrocautery and thereby protect against oversensing and spurious inhibition. Newer pacemakers may exhibit a variety of responses to placing a magnet over the pulse generator—although continuous asynchronous pacing is still the commonest response, some devices only deliver a brief period of asynchronous pacing for diagnostic testing and others no effect at all. With widespread uptake of noise-reversion modes, the need for magnet activation has been substantially reduced.

The response of an ICD to magnet placement depends on the model and programmed settings. Usually magnet activation will inhibit delivery of all tachycardia therapies without affecting anti-bradycardia pacing while the magnet is over the pulse generator, but the ICD becomes fully active again as soon as it is removed. In practice, the vast majority of ICDs (> 95%) are configured in this way. Certain manufacturers offer the possibility of deactivating therapies by a brief application of the magnet (20–30s) usually signalled by beeping tones; the device must then be reactivated by another magnet application. Rarely, the magnet response of the ICD may have been programmed off altogether.

# Preoperative assessment

Prior to all elective procedures in patients with pacemakers or ICDs, the surgical team should liaise with the supervising cardiologist/clinic to establish the following.

- Nature of the device (bradycardia pacemaker, ICD, CRT device, etc.), the manufacturer, and model.
- Date of implant and indication.
- Current device status and settings.
- If the last routine check was within the preceding 3–6 months and confirmed normal function, battery, and lead status, re-evaluation is not necessary. Otherwise, a further interrogation prior to surgery may be advisable (further checks may be needed if the device is subject to a manufacturer or regulatory safety advisory notice).
- Degree of pacemaker dependency and appropriate strategy to guard against the risk of asystole in high-risk cases (see below).
- In ICD patients, agree the strategy for avoiding inappropriate detection and tachyarrhythmia therapies during surgery, either programming the device to 'monitor only' mode temporarily or by application of a magnet to disable therapies.
- General cardiac condition, bearing in mind that most ICD patients have advanced heart disease and complex medication regimes.

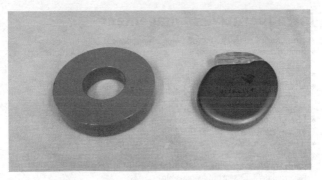

**Fig. 17.1** Medical grade pacemaker ring magnet shown next to an ICD.

# Intraoperative management

At the time of surgery, the following precautions should be observed.
- Ensure availability of cardiopulmonary resuscitation equipment and temporary external/transvenous pacing.
- Continuous ECG monitoring throughout.
- Use of an alternative method of pulse detection, either pulse oximetry or intra-arterial pressure monitoring, in case the ECG monitor is obscured by electrical noise during diathermy.
- Use of bipolar diathermy wherever possible, preferably in short, intermittent bursts and at the lowest effective output.
- If monopolar diathermy/electrocautery is unavoidable, ensure that the cutaneous return electrode is positioned so as to keep the current pathway (diathermy electrode to the patch) as far away from the pacemaker/ICD system as possible.
- For patients at high risk of asystole (i.e. pacemaker-dependent), consider reprogramming to asynchronous mode intraoperatively or use of a magnet (if appropriate model), and/or precautionary placement of transcutaneous electrodes for temporary external pacing support.
- For ICD patients, ensure deactivation of tachyarrhythmia therapies during the procedure as previously agreed with the patient's cardiologist. Ideally, this would involve formal reprogramming of the device into a 'monitor only' mode beforehand and then reactivation of the tachycardia therapies prior to leaving the operating theatre. In practice, personnel/logistic restrictions often mean that a ring magnet over the pulse generator (carefully secured) is used to disable therapies. This is the commonest approach and it is usually completely effective. The magnet should be removed before the patient is sent to the recovery area.
- While the ICD is deactivated, the patient must be continuously monitored for ventricular tachyarrhythmias, which need to be treated conventionally (or, if a magnet is being used, the device may be reactivated by removing it). In high-risk cases, consideration should be given to precautionary placement of external defibrillation pads particularly if there may be difficulty gaining access to the anterior chest wall without compromising the surgical field.

**Emergency surgery**

- As far as possible the precautions outlined in the section on intraoperative management should be followed.
- In this setting, there is usually no choice but to rely on magnet deactivation of ICD therapies with the same caveat about the need for monitoring and back-up external defibrillation.
- Similarly, clinical magnets can be used in pacemaker patients to induce asynchronous pacing in the unlikely event that electrocautery causes spurious inhibition/significant bradycardia, accepting that this will not work in a proportion of cases.
- Very rarely, it may be necessary to fall back on temporary transcutaneous or even transvenous pacing (📖 p. 155) if the use of electrocautery cannot be avoided but causes asystole in pacing-dependent cases despite the measures outlined previously.
- Where it has not been possible to assess pacemaker/ICD function preoperatively (applies to most emergency cases), contact should be made with the cardiology team as soon as possible afterwards and, where appropriate, formal interrogation and check of device function arranged.

## Postoperative management

- It is essential that all ICD functions that have been disabled are reactivated upon leaving the operating theatre.
- Any changes in pacing mode should be returned to their original settings, particularly if the device has been set to asynchronous pacing.
- If there has been any suggestion of malfunction during the perioperative period, then a full interrogation and check of the device parameters should be arranged as soon as possible, but otherwise this is not routinely required.
- Occasionally, reprogramming may be needed to deal with postoperative haemodynamic or arrhythmic problems, e.g. a temporary period of DDD pacing at higher rate to offset hypotension.

# Index